Mail this card today to stay up-to-date with the latest on Smart Drugs & Nutrients.

Name: _____

Address:_____

City:_____

State: _____ Zip: _____

Phone#: _____

Send a SASE for a list of physicians knowledgeable about smart drugs & nutrients. (Physicians: Please send your name, address, and short description of your practice to be added to our list.)

Would you like a Smart Drugs & Nutrients newsletter? ___

Please tell us what needs you have in this field that are not being met.

_____

_____

Please let us know about your experiences with smart drugs & nutrients. This information will help us keep our readers better informed (use a separate sheet if necessary.)

Comments: _____

_____

_____

Copy this page and mail it to B&J Publications, PO Box 2515-HC, Menlo Park, CA 94026, to stay up-to-date with the latest on **Smart Drugs & Nutrients**.

Name: _____

Address:_____

City:_____

State: _____ Zip: _____

Phone#: _____

Send a SASE for a list of physicians knowledgeable about smart drugs & nutrients. (Physicians: Please send your name, address, and short description of your practice to be added to our list.)

Would you like a Smart Drugs & Nutrients newsletter? ___

Please tell us what needs you have in this field that are not being met.

_____

_____

Please let us know about your experiences with smart drugs & nutrients. This information will help us keep our readers better informed (use a separate sheet if necessary.)

Comments: _____

_____

_____

What Others Are Saying About
Smart Drugs & Nutrients

"Smart Drugs & Nutrients is an excellent introduction to the field of cognition-enhancing compounds. It is also well-written and will be easily understood, even by people who do not have specific training in medicine."

Giacomo Spignoli, M.D., Ph.D.,
Pharmacology Research Director, L.Manetti-H.Roberts & Co.

"I'll not go down without a fight! Smart Drugs & Nutrients by Dean and Morgenthaler opens up the new world of nootropics - mind molecular support - that I know I need to explore personally; my father died of Alzheimer's."

Ernest Lawrence Rossi, Ph.D.

"This is a very important book. Very interesting and well documented...it is an absolutely essential and important subject."

Timothy Leary, Ph.D.

"An easy book to read and very interesting. I recommend it to any consumer who wants to be better informed and take more control over his or her own health."

Cliff Wong, R.Ph.

"I've never seen all this information together in one place before. The information is nicely summarized and well organized. Smart Drugs & Nutrients is a wonderful self-help manual because of the documentation of sources for both the substances and more information. I was especially pleased with the section regarding these smart drugs and the law. Physicians wanting to prescribe these drugs will find this section very useful."

Robert Buckley, M.D.

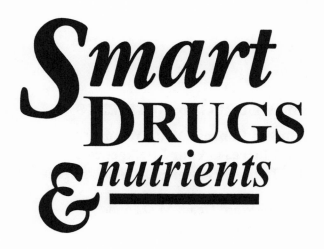

Smart DRUGS & *nutrients*

*How To Improve Your Memory
and Increase Your Intelligence
Using the Latest Discoveries in Neuroscience*

by
Ward Dean, M.D.
and
John Morgenthaler

B&J Publications — Santa Cruz, CA

SMART DRUGS & NUTRIENTS

How to Improve Your Memory
and Increase Your Intelligence
Using the Latest Discoveries in Neuroscience

By Ward Dean, M.D., and
John Morgenthaler

Published by:
B&J Publications
P.O. Box 2515-HC
Menlo Park, CA 94026

Printed by Instant Improvement, Inc. with the permission of B&J Publications. For information, address Instant Improvement, Inc., 210 East 86th Street, New York, New York 10028.

Sixth Printing 1991

First Hardcover Printing 1992

Printed in the United States of America

Library of Congress Catalog Card Number: 90-84066

Ward Dean, M.D., and John Morgenthaler
SMART DRUGS & NUTRIENTS: How To Improve Your Memory and Increase Your Intelligence Using the Latest Discoveries in Neuroscience
First Edition
ISBN 0-941683-24-9 Hardcover

Table of Contents

Acknowledgements

Special thanks go to all of the following individuals:
William Powell and Burl T. Moss for their crucial roles in creating and editing this book, Cathi Marsh for fantastic graphics, Gregory Bennett for the super photographs, and Hilary Hamm for marvelous business management.

We would also like to thank:

Deborah Benner, Sally Binford, Ph.D., Bob Buckley, M.D., Rue Burlingham, Dede Callichy, Jeffrey Devon Card, Sunah Cherwin, Paul Clark for his help collecting graphics materials, Kris Dean, Kumja Dean, Nancy Denenberg, Beverly DesChaux, Magi Discoe, Laura Fast, Amanita Faust, Steven Wm. Fowkes, Nancy Frank, John Furber, Ken Goffman, Ira Goldberg, Deborah Hart, Michael Hutchison, Mike Hyson, Ph.D., John S. James, Richard Kaufman, Ph.D., Alison Kennedy, Gimli Klein, Gerald Larson, Pat, Fred, and Wayne Morgenthaler, Ethel Neal, Scott Paddor, Durk Pearson and Sandy Shaw for their encouragement and help, Ross Pelton, R.Ph., Ph.D., and Taffy Clarke Pelton for their inspiration and hard work, Judy Pincus, Curtis Ponzi, Betty Powell, Dan Poynter, William Regelson, M.D., for his work on DHEA, Mark Rennie, Michael Rosenbaum, M.D., Sandoz Pharmaceuticals, Diane Smith, James South, Giacomo Spignoli, M.D., for providing much of the section on pyroglutamate and lots of help and advice, Arnold Stillman, Robert THK Trossel, M.D., UCB Pharmaceuticals, Jim Warshauer, Julie Weber, and Cricket Wingfield, M.D.

Disclaimer

This book is not intended to provide medical advice. It is intended to be educational and informational only.

Although most of the substances discussed in this book are remarkably free from adverse side effects, combinations of these substances alone or with other nutrients or drugs you may be taking may have unknown adverse effects. We recommend consulting with a knowledgeable physician before embarking on a cognition enhancement program of your own design.

Introduction

Science is changing our understanding of the human brain and of human intelligence. There is a whole new concept of what intelligence is and why some people are more intelligent than others. Scientists no longer believe that our intelligence is determined strictly by genetics. The concept of a fixed intelligence is a limiting belief and turns out to be untrue. Now we know that you can develop and increase your intelligence.

There is good reason to do so.

As we are exposed to a world of constantly increasing complexity and competition, faced with the information explosion and sensory overload, memory sharpness and increased thinking ability become imperative. People no longer do the same job for their entire lives. Many career paths require that people continue to educate themselves. Some professions require regular testing to establish that professional people are staying abreast of new developments. A corporation may be structured so that employees must compete intellectually for promotions and raises. The competition in these situations is every bit as real and intense as the competition on the playing fields. We believe that more and more business people and scholars are looking for the kind of "edge" that athletes get from science.

Science tells us that you can increase your intellectual abilities when you practice mental exercises (Bandler, 1985), when you do certain sensorimotor exercises (Ayres, 1989, Feldenkrais, 1985), or if you live in an enriched environment (Diamond, 1988). Research also shows that you may increase your intelligence by taking certain substances that have recently been shown to improve learning, memory, and concentration.

This book is an introductory guide to the use of this exciting new technology: drugs and nutrients that can increase your brain power and improve your memory, concentration, and ability to learn. There are dozens of substances that have been demonstrated to improve animal and human intelligence. In this book we present a practical guide as to how the most widely tested and potentially beneficial of these substances are being used.

We describe how others have used these smart drugs and nutrients for improved exam-taking ability, better job performance and increased productivity. We cover their use in delaying age-related intelligence decrease (including dealing with senility), and helping to deal with memory problems resulting from alcohol, tobacco, or drug abuse.

Our book is organized so that you can easily decide which of the drugs and nutrients might be of interest. The index can be used to look up symptoms or complaints as a quick way of finding smart drugs and nutrients of interest to you. For example, if you have a problem with fatigue, you can look that up in the index to find sections which might help you.

Some of the effects which have been reported from taking smart drugs and nutrients include:

1. Increased alertness, mental energy, and concentration.
2. Increased ability to concentrate for longer periods of time.
3. Increased ability to memorize material.
4. Greater productivity, organization, and planning ability.
5. Improved verbal memory.
6. Improved problem-solving ability.
7. Alleviation of depression.
8. Improved overall health.
9. Improved sexual performance.

If you are planning to use any of the smart drugs and nutrients we discuss to assist you in taking tests or examinations, we suggest that you carefully read the section titled The Use of Cerebroactive Substances. In addition, we strongly recommend that you consult a qualified physician before using smart drugs.

Some of the substances we write about can be obtained from your health food store. Others must be prescribed by a physician, and some of the newer, most effective smart drugs are only available overseas. In Appendix A (see page 165) we list some overseas mail-order sources for many of these compounds. We also have included some so new that they are not yet commercially available.

Smart Drugs & Nutrients will be useful to virtually anyone who uses their brain. Physicians who practice preventive medicine or who treat patients with memory or other neurological disorders will benefit from it, as it contains information that is not readily available elsewhere.

Finding A Physician

We urge anyone who wants to use smart drugs to do so under the supervision of a physician. Unfortunately, in our current legal climate, many physicians are unwilling to venture beyond the narrow limits of their training. Some physicians will discourage the experimental use of cognition-enhancing substances, regardless of their overwhelming record of safety.

If your physician is not aware of the potential of smart drugs, and is not willing to investigate this new science, we recommend that you contact the American College of Advancement in Medicine (ACAM) or the Huxley Institute for Biosocial Research for the name of a physician in your area. ACAM's number is (714) 583 7666 or (800) 532 3688. The Huxley Institute's number is (407) 393 6167 or (800) 847 3802. These physicians are among the most innovative physician-scientists in the world, and can probably provide you with appropriate guidance.

We also recommend that you fill out the yellow reader-response card at the front of this book and send it to us along with a self-addressed stamped envelope so we can send you our own list of physicians knowledgeable about smart drugs. (Physicians: please send your name, address, and a short description of your practice to be added to our list.) We will keep your address on file to keep you informed about additions to our directory of physicians, new editions of this book, and new resources for intelligence enhancement.

Sharing Knowledge

This field of research is exploding. We know that we have not been able to find all of the important intelligence increasing materials. We know that even though we searched the largest computer database in the world, we have missed some important data about the substances we do write about. If we have left out a drug or nutrient that you know increases intelligence, or if we have overlooked critical data about the cerebroactive materials included in this book, please write to us as soon as possible with your experiences or references.

We would also like to hear about your experiences with smart drugs and nutrients. This information will help us keep our readers better informed. The yellow reader response card at the front of this book has space for your comments, or you can send us a letter outlining your experiences. You can write to us care of:

B&J Publications
P.O. Box 2515-HC
Menlo Park, CA 94026

We look forward to hearing from you.

Age-Related Mental Decline

In other countries, diseases such as Alzheimer's, Korsakoff's syndrome, organic brain syndrome, and non-Alzheimer's senility are treated with drugs that are not available here. Other substances that are available in the U.S. have shown some efficacy against these diseases, but doctors here may be unfamiliar with the research.

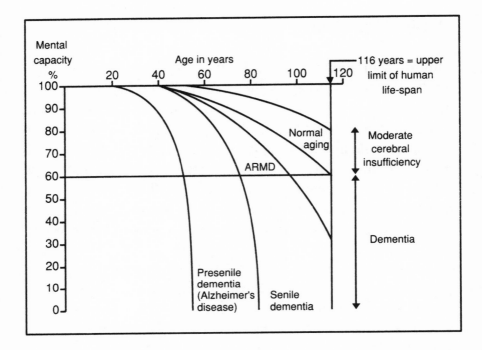

Decline of mental capacity with normal aging, age-related mental decline (ARMD), senile dementia, and Alzheimer's disease. (Redrawn from Age-Related Mental Decline and Dementias, The Place of Hydergine, Sandoz product literature booklet.)

At this time it is difficult to predict which people with senility will show positive results. In some of the studies we cite, individuals have exhibited remarkable improvement with a single drug or combination of drugs. We believe that individual biochemical differences may cause the inconsistency of results. In other words, each individual showing signs of senility may respond to a unique combination of drugs. Although shotgun-type drug combinations may be beneficial for one person, the same combination might adversely affect someone else. Thus, it is essential to work with a knowledgeable physician. Use this book's index and the section titled The Use of Cerebroactive Substances to custom-design a combination drug program for the person with senility. Start as soon as possible. The sooner the treatment is begun, the greater is the likelihood of beneficial results.

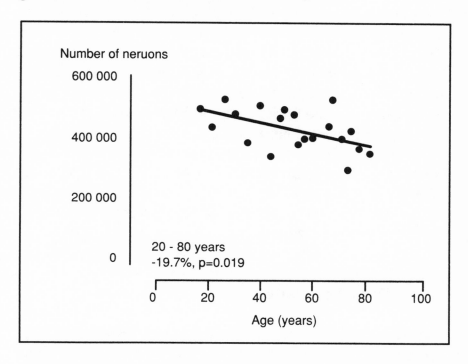

*Age-related decrease in the number of neurons in the olivary nucleus of the brain stem in humans. (Redrawn from **Age-Related Mental Decline and Dementias, The Place of Hydergine,** Sandoz product literature booklet.)*

Recreational Drugs and Mental Decline

Regular users of alcohol, cigarettes, and other recreational drugs such as cocaine or marijuana often complain of declining mental functioning. Alcoholics and pot users often have problems with short-term memory loss. Cigarettes also adversely affect mental functioning by greatly reducing the oxygen supply to the brain by causing not only short-term vasoconstriction, but also by tying up red blood cells with carbon monoxide (greatly reducing the oxygen capacity of the blood). This leads to premature atherosclerosis, as well as a compensatory increase in the number of red blood cells. This causes "thicker" blood, further worsening blood flow and oxygen delivery. Cocaine abusers often lose their ability to concentrate. This is particularly ironic since many people begin using cocaine for its ability to help the user concentrate for long periods of time. Chronic abuse, however, brings on paradoxical effects. The drugs and nutrients listed in this book can be of great help in combatting the deleterious effects of "recreational" drugs. However, we strongly discourage the use of illegal or legal recreational drugs, including coffee, cigarettes, and alcohol.

Smart Drug Newsletter

You can keep your finger on the pulse of new smart drugs research by subscribing to *Smart Drug News*, a newsletter published by the Cognition Research Enhancement Institute (CERI). You'll find more information about the newsletter in Appendix E of this book on page 185.

About The Scientific References

Every assertion we make in this book is based on scientific research. We have provided references to this scientific literature throughout this book so that you may review the original research. However, to avoid disrupting the flow of text we deviate slightly from scientific editorial conventions. When we refer to a research paper in the text, we give only the first author's name and year of publication. The complete reference, with all authors, is given at the end of each chapter.

References:

Ayres, J. **Sensory Integration**. Los Angeles: Western Psychological Services, 1989.

Bandler, R. **Using Your Brain For A Change**. Moab, Utah: Real People Press, 1985.

Diamond, M. **Enriching Heredity**. New York: The Free Press, 1988.

Feldenkrais, M. **The Potent Self: A Guide To Spontaneity**. San Francisco: Harper & Row, 1985.

Is All This Legal?

The fact that there are effective smart drugs and nutrients being manufactured today is good news. It is even better news that they can be purchased legally. How this is done, and what complications or qualifications may enter into such purchases is what this section is about.

Over-The-Counter Cognition Enhancement

First, the easy part. Some of the compounds we write about can be purchased over-the-counter from any source that specializes in the sale of nutritional supplements, including the sources we list in Appendix A (see page 165).

FDA Approved Drugs

Other compounds listed are FDA-approved drugs and can be purchased in this country with a prescription. It is important to understand, however, what "approved" and "unapproved" mean in FDA terminology. Under the Federal Food, Drug, and Cosmetic (FD&C) Act, a drug approved for marketing may be labeled, promoted, and advertised by the manufacturer only for those uses for which the drug's safety and effectiveness have been established, and which the FDA has approved. These are commonly referred to as "approved uses." This means that adequate and well-controlled clinical trials have documented these uses, and the results of the trials have been reviewed and approved by the FDA.

It is important to know that the FDA has no category for drugs that improve cognition in normal, healthy people. If a drug is to be approved at all, it must be approved for the treatment of a known disease such as Alzheimer's disease, multiple-infarct dementia, or senility.

There are many drugs that are both safe and effective which are not approved for use in the U.S. Sometimes it is because the pharmaceutical company knows that it simply could not make a profit after going through the extraordinarily expensive and lengthy process required to obtain FDA approval. Another reason drugs might not receive approval is that pharmaceutical companies have little interest in working on any drug that cannot be patented. There are several natural compounds (such as choline) discussed in this book which have cognitive enhancing effects. But no one can patent a natural compound. Without a patent, the pharmaceutical company that spends the money to get FDA approval for a drug will then have to compete with other pharmaceutical companies who did not spend the approval money, but can now sell the approved drug.

Physicians should be aware that by FDA law they have the right to prescribe any medication they believe will be helpful to their patient. It does not matter if the prescription represents a use for the drug that is not the FDA approved use.

Physicians are often reluctant to prescribe drugs for cognitive enhancement since it is not an "approved use". In April, 1982, the FDA issued a bulletin which included an important policy statement. The statement clarified the questions about prescribing drugs for "unapproved" uses, stating that physicians may prescribe drugs for unapproved uses in order to provide the best possible health care to the American public. The bulletin clearly stated that the use of "approved" drugs for "unapproved" uses is not only legal, but is one of the primary means of therapeutic innovation. It also said that, "valid new uses for drugs already on the market are often first discovered through serendipitous observations and therapeutic innovation." The term "unapproved uses" is misleading. It would appear that the FDA approves of the use of drugs for "unapproved" uses. Please see Appendix F for a reprint of this section of the April, 1982 issue of the FDA Drug Bulletin.

Overseas Drugs By Mail

The physician also has the right to prescribe drugs which have not been approved for any use in the U.S. Also, although it is not widely known, a July, 1988 FDA ruling now makes it quite legal for individuals to import effective drugs used elsewhere but not available in the U.S. The importation and mail shipment of a three-month supply of medications, for personal use, is now legal as long as they are regarded as safe in other countries. The new ruling, FDA Pilot Guidelines Chapter 971, was made as a result of heavy pressure from AIDS political action groups, which insisted that AIDS sufferers were denied access to potentially life-saving substances that were widely used abroad but were still unapproved for use in the U.S. You will find the text of these new FDA guidelines in Appendix G.

News of the FDA's policy change appeared in the New York

Times as follows:

F.D.A. EXPANDS EARLIER STAND BY ALLOW-
ING MAILING OF DRUGS

WASHINGTON, July 25 — When the Food and Drug Administration announced on Saturday that it would allow Americans to import unapproved drugs from abroad in small quantities, it was formalizing its longstanding practice of looking the other way when travelers brought back foreign drugs.

More significantly, it also stated for the first time that it would permit routine mail shipments of such drugs, making them potentially available to vastly more people than the few who venture abroad in search of treatments.

Certainly, both officials and critics agree that timely completion of human trials of potential drugs to determine which are truly effective is more important in the long run than the importation of unproved drugs. Despite recent pledges by officials from the F.D.A. and the National Institutes of Health to speed up the process of drug evaluation, there remains a wide gap in perceptions about the realistic chances of finding useful treatments soon.

The new policy was the direct result of pressure from desperate AIDS patients, who have only one approved treatment available in the country, AZT, or azidothymidine, which is too toxic for many patients to take for long periods...

In cases where overseas shipments are stopped by U.S. Customs (which should be rare), the recipient will be sent a standard form letter and will have to sign a statement stating that the drug is for their personal use, and also to provide the government with the name of the physician responsible for his or her treatment with the product in the shipment.

The FDA has made it clear, however, that it will not tolerate "commercial promotion" of unapproved drugs to U.S. citizens by overseas companies taking unfair advantage of the situation to promote unproven drugs to people in the U.S.

There are no guarantees that the FDA will not change its mind about the mail importation policy and act to reverse it. But at the time of this writing this is how the law and FDA policy stand. We have provided a list of mail-order sources in Appendix A (see page 165). We hope that the overseas companies listed will have the good sense to comply with all FDA regulations, i.e., supplying only items which have been proven to be safe and have no abuse potential, and not commercializing their services (which we take to mean they must not advertise but merely supply to informed individuals). This will decrease the chances that there could be FDA action against them.

References:

Anderson, K., Anderson, L. **Orphan Drugs**. Los Angeles, CA: The
        Body Press, 1987, pp. VIII-XXVI.
Boffey, P.M., **New York Times**. July 25, 1988.
Food And Drug Administration. **FDA Drug Bulletin**. April 1982.
Food And Drug Administration. **Regulatory Procedures Manual**.
        Chapter 9-71.
James, J.S., **AIDS Treatment News**. July 29, 1988, Number 61, pp.
        1-4.
Pelton, R., Pelton, T.C. **Mind Food & Smart Pills**. New York: Double-
        day, 1989.

The Use of Cerebroactive Compounds

Although most of the smart drugs and nutrients discussed in this book are remarkably free from adverse side effects, combinations of these substances alone or with other nutrients or drugs may have unknown adverse effects. We recommend consulting a knowledgeable physician before embarking on a cognition-enhancing program.

If you are going to experiment with any of these compounds, we recommend that you add only one at a time to your smart drug regimen. This is the only way you will be able to distinguish the effects of the compounds.

Although we discuss dosage ranges for each of the smart drugs and nutrients, please think of these dosages as general guidelines. The dosages here have been derived for the "average" person, based on statistical findings in the research. However, you are not average. Each person's biochemistry is unique, and only you can determine how much of each compound is optimal for you. Studies show that for any particular compound, an optimum dosage may vary from person to person by as much as 20 times.

Remember Goldilocks? Well, the key to using cognition enhancers is to find the dose that's not too much and not too little, but "just right."

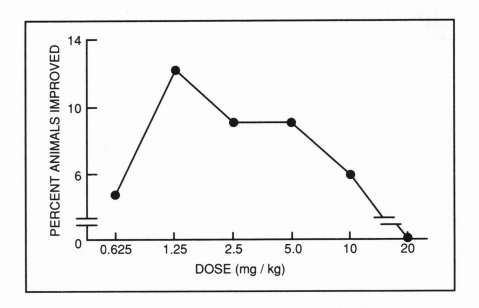

Facilitation of short-term memory in rats with pramiracetam. (Redrawn from Poschel, 1983.)

"A bell-shaped dose-effect relationship is a typical feature of all drugs acting on cognitive processes" (Pepeu, 1989). The graph above is an example of a bell-shaped dose response curve for pramiracetam. This means that for each compound there is an optimum dose, and above or below this dosage, the effects are not as profound. The same is probably true for most of the smart drugs and nutrients discussed in this book. Furthermore, excessively high doses of some compounds may actually produce reverse effects (Heiby, 1989).

Kenneth and Lois Anderson write in their excellent book, *Orphan Drugs*, "An effective individual dosage is often established in the same way that one makes an individual adjustment in the amount of coffee or tea consumed during the day—by the trial-and-error technique sometimes called titration. Most people learn through experience to estimate the amount of coffee or tea they can consume without discomfort and adjust their daily caffeine beverage intake accordingly. The same process works for many medications."

Subtle or even major improvements in cognitive function can sometimes go unnoticed. One way to measure changes in your own cognitive abilities is to ask your friends and family. Tell them you are experimenting with some new technologies and you would like them to watch you a little more closely. This will get you a more objective measurement than you could get on your own.

When using smart drugs and nutrients pay particular attention to changes in any of the following: alertness, mental energy, concentration, being able to concentrate for longer periods at a time, ability to memorize material, productivity, organization, planning ability, verbal memory, problem-solving ability, mood, sexual desire, overall health, and performance at intellectual games such as chess or computer games.

Synergy

In one fascinating study, a team of researchers led by Raymond Bartus (1981) administered the cognition enhancers choline and piracetam to a strain of aged lab rats noted for their age-related memory decline. "Those subjects given only choline (100 mg/kg) did not differ on the behavioral task from control animals administered vehicle (placebo). Rats given piracetam (100 mg/kg) performed slightly better than control rats ... but rats given the piracetam/choline combination (100 mg/kg of each) exhibited retention scores several times better than those given piracetam alone. In a second study it was shown that twice the dose of piracetam (200

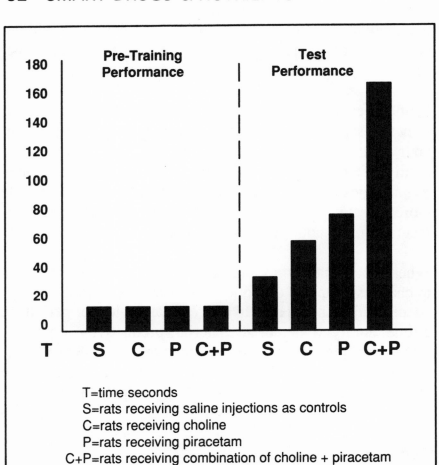

T=time seconds
S=rats receiving saline injections as controls
C=rats receiving choline
P=rats receiving piracetam
C+P=rats receiving combination of choline + piracetam

Rats placed in a box with a lighted chamber and dark chamber will normally prefer to go into the dark chamber. In this study these aged rats took less than 20 seconds to enter the dark chamber on the pre-training performance. Upon entry to the dark chamber the rats were subjected to mild foot shock. Twenty-four hours later the rats were returned to the box and tested for the length of time before they entered the dark chamber. Rats treated with either choline or piracetam took only slightly longer than controls to enter the dark chamber where they had previously received a shock, whereas rats treated with both choline and piracetam took nearly three times as long to enter the dark chamber. This indicates the rats' memory for the shock avoidance was greatly improved. (Redrawn from Bartus, 1981.)

mg/kg) or choline (200 mg/kg) alone, still did not enhance retention nearly as well as when piracetam and choline (100 mg/kg of each) were administered together." This is synergy, a process commonly found in nature where the whole is greater than the sum of the parts (Fuller, 1975).

One mouse model study found that combining two memory-increasing drugs allowed for a reduction in the optimal dose by 66.2% to as much as 95.7% (Flood, 1985). Another, similar, study conducted by the same team found 95% reduction in optimal dosages when two drugs were combined (Flood, 1983).

These studies and the ones we cite below were published by Flood and the late Arthur Cherkin. Cherkin, a prolific drug researcher, told us about an unpublished mouse experiment he conducted combining piracetam with Hydergine. His results indicated that the optimal dose of this combination could be 5 times less than the optimal dosage of each when used alone.

The good news here is that taking Hydergine and piracetam together may be far less expensive than taking either alone. However, you must still ascertain the optimum dose for yourself as per our previous instructions.

Taking Exams

If you are planning to use any of the smart drugs and nutrients we have discussed to assist you in taking tests or examinations, we suggest that you follow some rules.

Make certain that the substances you are using actually make you smarter. If possible, purchase a workbook for the test you intend to take. Take a sample test without the substances, then take another sample test with them. Do this several times to be certain that you do feel smarter, think more clearly, and do better on the test with your choice of smart drugs and nutrients.

Remember that more is not necessarily better. Use the information in the rest of this section to ascertain the optimum substance or combination of substances and their correct dosages.

Beware of potential problems. For example, you might choose to take Inderal one and a half hours before a test in order to avoid having a fear response during the testing. Although it is generally well tolerated, propranolol (Inderal) can cause nausea if taken on an empty stomach, especially with black coffee. Read the precautions we include for each drug.

The research we've seen suggests that coffee may have some *intelligence-lowering effects*. Unless you are truly addicted and require coffee for functioning, we recommend that coffee be avoided during intellectually-demanding situations.

If you become familiar with the range of compounds available, you will be able to choose among them for different uses. A perfect example is vasopressin. One quick inhalation of vasopressin can clear your head and sharpen your recall in ten seconds. This can be invaluable for situations where you are required to be your sharpest on a moment's notice.

Other smart drugs, such as piracetam, will make learning new material much easier. Smart drugs are most useful if you experiment and find out which ones work for you.

References:

Anderson, K., Anderson, L. **Orphan Drugs**. Los Angeles, CA: The Body Press, 1987, p. 132.

Bartus, R.T., Dean R.L. 3d, Sherman, K.A., Friedman, E., Beer, B. "Profound Effects of Combining Choline and Piracetam on Memory Enhancement and Cholinergic Function in Aged Rats." **Neurobiology of Aging**. 1981, Vol. 2, pp. 105-11.

Berga, P., Beckett, P.R., Roberts, D.J., Llenas, J., Massingham, R. "Synergistic Interactions Between Piracetam and Dihydro-ergocristine in Some Animal Models of Cerebral Hypoxia and Ischaemia." **Arzneimittelforschung**. 1986, 36 (9), pp. 1314-20.

Ferris, S.H., et al. "Combination of Choline/Piracetam in the Treatment of Senile Dementia." **Psychopharmacology Bulletin**. 1982, Vol. 18, pp. 94-98.

Flood, J.F., Smith, G.E., Cherkin, A. "Memory Retention: Potentiation of Cholinergic Drug Combinations in Mice." **Neurobiology of Aging**. 1983, 4 (1) pp. 37-43.

Flood, J.F., Smith, G.E., Cherkin, A. "Memory Enhancement: Supra-Additive Effect of Subcutaneous Cholinergic Drug Combinations in Mice." **Psychopharmacology**. 1985, 86 (1-2) pp. 61-7.

Flood, J.F., Cherkin, A. "Effect of Acute Arecoline, Tacrine and Arecoline + Tacrine Post-Training Administration on Retention in Old Mice." **Neurobiology of Aging**. 1988, 9 (1) pp. 5-8.

Flood, J.F., Smith, G.E., Cherkin, A. "Two-Drug Combinations of Memory Enhancers: Effect of Dose Ratio Upon Potency and Therapeutic Window, in Mice." **Life Science**. 1988, 42 (21) pp. 2145-54.

Friedman, E., Sherman, K.A., Ferris, S.H., Reisberg, B., Bartus, R.T., Schneck, M.K. "Clinical Response to Choline Plus Piracetam in Senile Dementia: Relation to Red-Cell Choline Levels." **The New England Journal of Medicine**. 1981, 304, No. 24, pp. 1490-91.

Fuller, R.B. **Synergetics**. New York: Macmillan Publishing, 1975.

Heiby, W. **The Reverse Effect**. Deerfield, IL: Mediscience

Pepeu, G., Spignoli, G., Giovannini, M.G., Magnani, M. "The Relationship Between the Behavioral Effects of Cognition-Enhancing Drugs and Brain Acetylcholine. Nootropic Drugs and Brain Acetylcholine." **Pharmacopsychiatry**. 1989, 22 Supplement 2, pp. 116-9.

Poschel, B.P.H., Marriott, J.G., Gluckman, M.I. "Pharmacology of the Cognition Activator Pramiracetam (CI-879)." **Drugs Under Experimental and Clinical Research**. 1983, vol. 9(12), pp. 853-71.

Nootropics:
More Doctors Recommend

We are very excited about nootropics, a new class of smart drugs. We believe that this development is a major advance in neuroscience. The word nootropics was coined to describe substances that improve learning, memory consolidation, and memory retrieval without other central nervous system effects and with low toxicity, even at extremely high doses (Giurgea, 1972). Doctors prescribe nootropics to millions of people outside of the U.S. every year. Surprisingly, none of the nootropic drugs have been approved in the U.S. A number of companies are attempting or have attempted to receive approval from the FDA to sell newly-developed (and patented) nootropic drugs in the U.S., but so far without success. Most of the people we know who have tried nootropics such as piracetam have become die-hard fans (see Appendix D on page 179 for testimonials). The nootropics hold the most promise for people with Alzheimer's disease and other forms of senility.

Although there is some disagreement in the scientific community as to which substances are nootropics and which are not, we have included in this section drugs that are most often referred to as nootropics in the scientific literature.

Some Definitions

Before we begin to describe the uses and actions of the nootropics, let's look at some "brain basics" — including some terms we will be using frequently in this book.

Mental and physical functions are partly governed by a group of chemicals called neurotransmitters (Kaufman, 1986). These chemicals carry impulses (messages) between nerve cells. Some are part of the cholinergic system. This refers to the parts of the nervous system that use acetylcholine as a neurotransmitter.

Acetylcholine (ACh) plays an important role in memory and learning. It also controls sensory input signals and muscular control. ACh is a stimulatory neurotransmitter which, when released by muscle nerves, makes those muscles contract. Unfortunately, ACh production declines with age. This leads to a loss of cognitive functioning which may be counteracted or even prevented with the substances described in this book.

There are many other terms defined in the glossary in the back of this book.

Pyrrolidone Derivatives

The most intriguing nootropics are the pyrrolidone derivatives. This class includes piracetam and its analogues oxiracetam, pramiracetam, aniracetam, and some others. The mechanism by which these have such a remarkable memory-improvement effect is still uncertain. Most studies suggest these drugs work by affecting the cholinergic system in the brain, that is, the parts of the nervous system that use acetylcholine as a neurotransmitter.

Molecular structures of some of the piracetam-type nootropic drugs.

Some recent observations show that some interactions also take place with the adrenal cortex and are involved with adrenal steroid production. All four of these compounds are inactive in laboratory animals which have had their adrenal cortex removed or which have been treated with drugs that block the adrenal cortex. When we learn how these drugs work, we may also understand more about the basic processes of memory storage (Mondadori, 1989).

The nootropics generally have an "inverted U dose-response curve", which means that more is not necessarily better. If you decide to use nootropics, you must ascertain the optimum amount (see The Use of Cerebroactive Substances.) Combining two or more nootropics or other smart drugs and nutrients may also reduce the dose necessary for the optimum desired effects.

References:

Giurgea, C.E. "Pharmacology of Integrative Activity of the Brain. Attempt at Nootropic Concept in Psychopharmacology." **Actualites Pharmacologiques**. 1972, 25, pp. 115-56.

Giurgea, C.E. "The 'Nootropic' Approach to the Pharmacology of the Integrative Activity of the Brain." **Conditional Reflex**. 1973, Vol. 8, No. 2, pp. 108-15.

Giurgea, C.E. "A Drug for the Mind." **Chemtech**. June 1980, pp. 360-5.

Giurgea, C.E., Salama, M. "Nootropic Drugs." **Progress in Neuropsychopharmacology**. 1977, Vol. 1, pp. 235-47.

Kaufman, R. **The Age Reduction System**. New York: Rawson Associates 1986.

Mondadori, C. "The Effects of Nootropics on Memory: New Aspects for Basic Research." **Pharmacopsychiatry**. Oct 1989, 22 Supplement 2 pp. 102-6.

Nicholson, C. "Nootropics and Metabolically Active Compounds in

Alzheimer's Disease." **Biochemical Society Transactions**. 1989, 17(1) pp. 83-5

Pelton, R., Pelton, T.C. **Mind Food & Smart Pills**. New York: Doubleday, 1989.

Pepeu, G., Spignoli, G. Neurochemical Actions of "Nootropic Drugs". Advances in Neurology. Vol. 51: Alzheimer's Disease. Raven Press, Ltd., New York 1990.

Poschel, B.P.H. "New Pharmacologic Perspectives on Nootropic Drugs." **Handbook of Psychopharmacology**. 1988, pp. 11-18, pp. 24-25.

Piracetam (Nootropil)

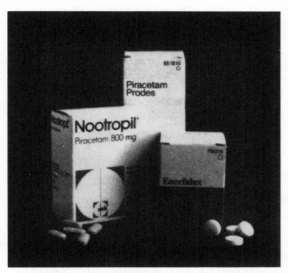

This drug is reported to be an intelligence-booster with no toxicity or addictive properties. Piracetam is inexpensive (under $0.85 per day) and available by mail (see Appendix A, page 165). The subjective effect described by some people is that piracetam "wakes up your brain." You'll find more personal accounts of the effects of this remarkable drug in the case histories and testimonials appendix (see page 179). Its effects and safety are so impressive that piracetam prompted the creation of a new pharmaceutical category called the nootropics.

The term nootropic comes from a Greek word meaning "acting on the mind". Since the invention of piracetam by UCB Laboratories in Belgium, other pharmaceutical companies have been scrambling to develop their own nootropics. Some of them being researched now include: vinpocetine, aniracetam, pramiracetam, and oxiracetam. As yet, there is no nootropic compound that is FDA-approved for sale in the U.S., but there is plenty of motivation on the part of pharmaceutical companies to get that approval. Financial analysts expect that the U.S. market for these smart drugs will soon be in excess of $1 billion per year (Pelton, 1989).

Piracetam is very similar in molecular structure to the amino acid pyroglutamate (see Pyroglutamate). Piracetam and pyroglutamate have the same "base" chemical structure, the 2-oxo-pyrrolidine, but they differ by the side chain. Pyroglutamate is 2-oxo-pyrrolidone carboxylic acid, and piracetam is 2-oxo-pyrrolidine acetamide.

Piracetam enhances cognition under conditions of hypoxia (too little oxygen), and also enhances memory and some kinds of learning in normal humans. Outside of the U.S., piracetam is used to treat alcoholism, stroke, vertigo, senile dementia, sickle-cell anemia, dyslexia, and numerous other health problems (Pelton, 1989).

One of the most intriguing effects of piracetam is that it promotes the flow of information between the right and left hemispheres of the brain (Buresova, 1976). We know that communication between the two sides of the brain is associated with flashes of creativity. This may also be the basis for piracetam's usefulness in the treatment of dyslexia (Dilanni, 1985).

The effect of piracetam may be increased if taken with DMAE, centrophenoxine, choline, or Hydergine. When choline and piracetam are taken together there is a synergistic effect that causes a greater improvement in memory than the sum of each when taken alone (Bartus, 1981).

We know of one person who claims she feels slightly agitated and depressed if she takes piracetam for more than a week without a choline supplement. This feeling is alleviated for her with a single dose of choline. It may be that the piracetam causes acetylcholine to be used up more quickly and that the choline helps to replace this important neurotransmitter.

One fascinating study suggests that piracetam might increase the number of cholinergic receptors in the brain. Older mice were given piracetam for two weeks and then the density of muscarinic cholinergic receptors in their frontal cortexes was measured. The researchers found that these older mice had 30-40% higher density of these receptors than before. (Pilch, 1988). Piracetam, unlike many other drugs, appears to have a regenerative effect on the nervous system.

One theory of Alzheimer's disease is that the decline of intellectual functions is partly caused by a decreased activity of the cholinergic system in the brain caused by cell death and cell degeneration. The researchers in the above study speculated that their findings could explain how piracetam works and could also explain the finding of Bartus and his colleagues regarding the profound effect of combining choline with piracetam on memory enhancement of old rats.

As mentioned previously, the late drug researcher Arthur Cherkin related to us that he believed the combination of Hydergine and piracetam potentiate each other up to five times. This highlights the importance of adjusting the dosages when multiple substances are taken because some of these substances will cause paradoxical effects when excessive amounts are taken.

Although piracetam is a derivative of GABA (Gamma Amino Butyric Acid, a neurotransmitter), there is no evidence that piracetam works through the GABAergic system. Some research even suggests GABA may inhibit memory and learning (Zhang, 1989).

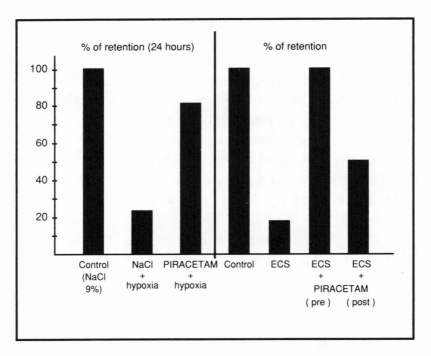

Piracetam protects rats from the memory-impairment effects of hypoxia and electroconvulsive seizure (ECS). In the first part of this study, rats are administered NaCl (saline) as a control, NaCl + hypoxia, or piracetam + hypoxia. In the second part, rats are administered no treatment (control), ECS, ECS + piracetam pre-treatment, or ECS + piracetam post-treatment. All of the control rats (100%) had memory retention of the training task at 24 hours. The percentage of rats with memory retention is severely reduced with hypoxia and ECS, and increased by the addition of piracetam. (Redrawn from Giurgea, 1973.)

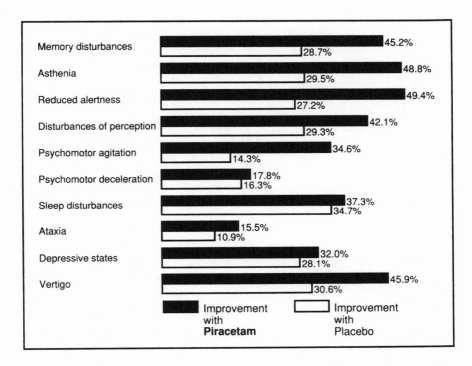

Percentage of improvement in symptoms of senile patients (average age of 67) given placebo or 2.4 gm per day of piracetam for only eight weeks in a double-blind study. (Redrawn from Nootropil in the Treatment of Early Symptoms of: Alzheimer's Disease, or Senile Dementia of Alzheimer Type, or Multi-Infarct Dementia, UCB Pharmaceutical Division.)

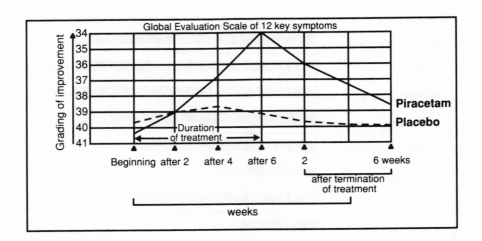

A double-blind controlled study in a group of patients with cerebral arteriosclerosis. All patients were scored on 15 parameters representative of disorders due to senility. Note that the piracetam group still shows improvement for weeks after termination of treatment. (Redrawn from Nootropil in the Treatment of Early Symptoms of: Alzheimer's Disease, or Senile Dementia of Alzheimer Type, or Multi-Infarct Dementia, UCB Pharmaceutical Division.)

Precautions: Piracetam may increase the effects of certain drugs, such as amphetamines, psychotropics, and Hydergine, as stated. Adverse effects are rare but include insomnia, psychomotor agitation, nausea, gastrointestinal distress, and headaches. Piracetam has virtually no known toxicity or contraindications.

Dosage: Piracetam is supplied in 400mg or 800mg capsules or tablets. The usual dose is 2400 to 4800 mg per day in three divided doses. Some literature recommends a high "attack" dose be taken for the first two days. We have noticed that often when people first take piracetam they do not notice any effect at all until they take a high dose (approximately 4000 to 8000mg). Thereafter, they may notice that a lower dosage is sufficient. Piracetam takes effect within 30 to 60 minutes.

Sources: Piracetam is not sold in the U.S. It can be purchased over the counter in Mexico or by mail from the sources listed in Appendix A (see page 165). Other names include: Avigilen, Cerebroforte, Cerebrospan, Cetam, Dinagen, Encefalux, Encetrop, Euvifor, Gabacet, Genogris, Memo-Puren, Nootron, Nootrop, Nootropil, Nootropyl, Normabrain, Norzetam, Novocetam, Pirroxil, Psycoton, Stimucortex, and UCB-6215.

References:

Anderson, K., Anderson, L. **Orphan Drugs**. Los Angeles, CA: The Body Press, 1987, p. 169.

Bartus, R.T., Dean R.L. 3d, Sherman, K.A., Friedman, E., Beer, B. "Profound Effects of Combining Choline and Piracetam on Memory Enhancement and Cholinergic Function in Aged Rats." **Neurobiology of Aging**. 1981, Vol. 2, pp. 105-11.

Buresova, O., Bures, J. "Piracetam-Induced Facilitation of Interhemispheric Transfer of Visual Information in Rats." **Psychopharmacologia**. 1976, Vol. 46, pp. 93-102.

Bylinsky, G. "Medicine's Next Marvel: The Memory Pill." **Fortune**. January 20, 1986, pp. 68-72.

Chase, C.H., Schmitt, R.L., Russel, G., Tallal, P. "A New Chemotherapeutic Investigation: Piracetam Effects on Dyslexia." **Annals of Dyslexia**. 1984, Vol. 34, pp. 29-48.

Conners, C.K., Blouin, A.G., Winglee, M., Lougee, L., O'Donnell, D., Smith, A. "Piracetam and Event-Related Potentials in Dyslexic Children." **Psychopharmacology Bulletin**. 1984, Vol. 20, pp. 667-73.

Dimond, S.J., Browers, E.Y.M. "Increase in the Power of Human Memory in Normal Man Through the Use of Drugs." **Psychopharmacology**. 1976, Vol. 49, pp. 307-9.

Dilanni, M., Wilsher, C.R., Blank, M.S., Conners, C.K., Chase, C.H.,

Funkenstein, H.H., Helfgott, E., Holmes, J.H., Lougee, L., Marletta, G.J., Milewski, J., Pirazzolo, F.J., Rudel, R.G., Tallal, P. "The Effects of Piracetam in Children with Dyslexia." **Journal of Clinical Psychopharmacology.** 1985, Vol. 5, pp. 272-8.

Donaldson, T. "Therapies to Improve Memory." **Anti-Aging News.** 1984, No. 4, pp. 13-21.

Ferris, S.H., et al. "Combination of Choline/Piracetam in the Treatment of Senile Dementia." **Psychopharmacology Bulletin.** 1982, Vol. 18, pp. 94-8.

Friedman, E., Sherman, K.A., Ferris, S.H., Reisberg, B., Bartus, R.T., Schneck, M.K. "Clinical Response to Choline Plus Piracetam in Senile Dementia: Relation to Red-Cell Choline Levels." **The New England Journal of Medicine.** 1981, 304, No. 24, pp. 1490-1.

Giurgea, C.E. "The 'Nootropic' Approach to the Pharmacology of the Integrative Activity of the Brain." **Conditional Reflex.** 1973, Vol. 8, No. 2, pp. 108-15.

Giurgea, C.E. "A Drug for the Mind." **Chemtech.** June 1980, pp. 360-65.

Giurgea, C.E., Salama, M. "Nootropic Drugs." **Progress in Neuropsychopharmacology.** 1977, Vol. 1, pp. 235-47.

Kent, S. "Piracetam Increases Brain Energy." **Anti-Aging News.** 1981, Vol. 2, No. 10, pp. 65-69.

Mindus, P., Cronholm, B., Levander, S.E., Schalling, D. "Piracetam--Induced Improvement of Mental Performance: A Controlled Study on Normally Aging Individuals." **ACTA Psychiatrica Scandinavia.** 1976, Vol. 54, pp. 150-60.

Mondadori, C., Classen, W., Borkowski, J., Ducret, T., Buerki, H., Schade, A. "Effects of Oxiracetam on Learning and Memory in Animals: Comparison with Piracetam." **Clinical Neuropharmacology.** 1986, Vol. 9, Supplement 13. New York: Raven Press, pp. S27-S37.

Nickerson, V.J., Wolthius, O.L. "Effect of the Acquisition-Enhancing Drug Piracetam on Rat Cerebral Energy Metabolism Comparison with Naftidrofuryl and Methamphetamine." **Biochemical Pharmacology.** 1976, Vol. 25, pp. 2241-4.

Parducz, A. "Depletion of Synaptic Vesicle Lipids in Stimulated Cholinergic Nerve Terminals." **Alzheimer's Disease: Advances in**

Basic Research and Therapies. Proceedings of the Third Meeting of the International Study Group of the Treatment of Memory Disorders Associated with Aging. Zurich, Switzerland, 1984, pp. 217-26.

Pearson, D., Shaw, S. **Durk Pearson & Sandy Shaw's Life Extension Newsletter.** October 1988, Vol 1, Number 8, p. 65.

Pellegata, R., et al. "Cyclic Gaba-Gabob Analogues." Presented at VI International meeting of the International Society For Neurochemistry, Copenhagen, August 21-26, 1977.

Pelton, R., Pelton, T.C. **Mind Food & Smart Pills.** New York: Doubleday, 1989.

Pepeu, G., and Spignoli, G. Neurochemical Actions of "Nootropic Drugs". **Advances in Neurology. Vol. 51: Alzheimer's Disease.** New York: Raven Press, Ltd., 1990.

Pilch, H., Muller, W.E. "Piracetam Elevates Muscarinic Cholinergic Receptor Density in the Frontal Cortex of Aged But Not of Young Mice." **Psychopharmacology.** 1988, 94, pp. 74-8.

Poschel, B.P.H. "New Pharmacologic Perspectives on Nootropic Drugs." **Handbook of Psychopharmacology.** 1988, pp. 11-18, pp. 24-5.

Stegink, A.J. "The Clinical Use of Piracetam, a New Nootropic Drug." **Arzneimittelforschung.** 1972, Vol. 22, No. 6, pp. 975-7.

U.C.B. Laboratories, Pharmaceutical Division. "Basic Scientific and Clinical Data of Nootropil." Brussels, Belgium: U.C.B. Laboratories, 1977.

Wilsher, C.R. "Piracetam and Dyslexia: Effects on Reading Tests." **Journal of Clinical Psychopharmacology.** 1987, Vol. 7, No. 4, pp. 230-7.

Wurtman, R.J., Magil, S.G., Reinstein, D.K. "Piracetam Diminishes Hippocampal Acetylcholine Levels in Rats." **Life Science.** 1981, Vol. 28, pp. 1091-3.

Zhang, S., et al. "Effects of Cerebral GABA Level on Learning and Memory." **Pharmacologica Sinica.** 1989 10(1): pp. 10-2.

Basle Reservor and Theramex. "Proceedings of the Third Meeting of the International Study Group of the Treatment of Memory Disorders Associated with Aging Zurich, Switzerland. 1984, pp. 237-40.

Pearson, D., Shaw, S. Durk Pearson & Sandy Shaw's Life Extension Newsletter. October 1986, vol 1, number 1, p 1-8.

Bellipanni, R. et al. "Dietic Interventions Analgesics." Presented at VI International meeting of the Association Society For Neurochemistry. Copenhagen, August 21-26, 1977.

Patton, P. Patton, T.C. Mind Food & Smart Pills. New York: Doubleday, 1991.

Pepeu, G., and Spignoli, G. "Nootropic Drugs and Nootropic Drugs" Advances in Neurology, vol 51, Alzheimer's Disease. New York: Raven Press, Inc. 1990.

Pilch, H., Muller, W.E. "Piracetam Elevates Muscarinic Cholinergic Receptor Density in the Frontal Cortex of Aged but Not of Young Mice." Psychopharmacology 1988, 94, pp. 74-8.

Poschel, B.P.H. "New Pharmacological Perspectives in Nootropic Drugs." Handbook of Psychopharmacology, vol 20, 1987, pp. 437-69, 204.

Singh, A.N. "The Effects of Piracetam." Journal of Geriatric Drugs. Aminoindaline therapy, 1977, vol 27, no. 2-3, pp. 973-7, 2-3.

U.S.R. Laboratories Information. "Deaner: Deaner Scientific and Clinical Data." The Complete Reference Program. U.S.R. Laboratories, 1977.

Wilson, C.R. "Reaction and Dysfunction after the Bleeding Level." Journal of Clinical Psychopharm macology 1981, Vol 7, no. 6, p. 23-27.

Weintraub, H.G., Mintzer, S.G., Ramjerra, P.L. "Premium Stimulants After month Anti-Stimul Lose in a Phase I conferences 1987 vol 56, no. 1654-7.

Zhang, G. et al. "Effects of Gossypol Acetate Level for Learning and Memory." Physiological Studies. 1989 1(1), pp. 104-5.

Aniracetam

Human studies have established that aniracetam is a powerful cognitive enhancer. Study participants improved their scores on a number of intelligence and memory tests (Saletu, 1980, 1984).

Aniracetam's chemical structure is similar to that of piracetam. Studies comparing the two found that aniracetam is effective in treating a wider range of problems than piracetam. Aniracetam is more powerful than piracetam.

In animal experiments, aniracetam has been shown to have a protective effect on the brain. Also, one study of 60 geriatric patients in a nursing home found that aniracetam had a significant "revitalizing" effect (Foltyn, 1983).

The mechanism of action of aniracetam is not known. It does not appear to act directly upon neurotransmitter systems such as GABA, catecholamines, serotonin or acetylcholine (Cumin, 1982).

Hoffmann-La Roche holds the U.S. patent on aniracetam. The corporation was attempting to gain FDA approval for Aniracetam, but has now assigned the rights to foreign firms. One Hoffmann-La Roche research department employee said that it is very difficult to meet the FDA's criteria for proving that a drug is effective for the treatment of Alzheimer's disease or senility.

Individuals we know who have experimented with aniracetam have described its effects as being very much like piracetam.

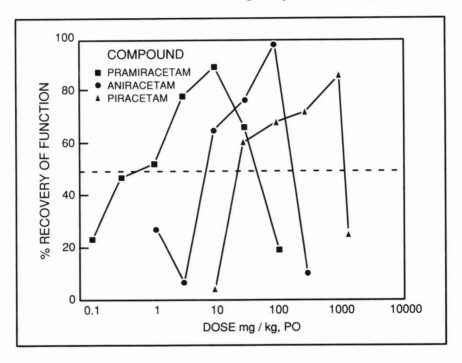

Three nootropic drugs protect mice from the memory disruption effects of electrobrain shock. (Redrawn from Gamzu, 1986.)

Precautions: Aniracetam has been tested in too few human studies to establish precautions. Preliminary findings indicate that, like other nootropics, it has little or no toxicity and few or no side effects.

Dosage: One study found that the maximum cognitive-enhancing effect occurred at 1000mg of aniracetam per day. Use of other smart drugs and nutrients concurrently will probably greatly reduce the optimum dosage.

Sources: Aniracetam is not approved for distribution in any country as far as we know. If it ever does become commercially available, U.S. doctors may be able to legally prescribe it for whatever uses they see fit. Overseas mail-order firms will probably offer aniracetam if it becomes available outside of the U.S. Other names for aniracetam include: Draganon, Ro 13-5057, and Sarpul.

References:

Cumin, R., Bandle, E.F., Gamzu, E., Haefely, W.E. "Effects of the Novel Compound Aniracetam (RO13-5057) Upon Impaired Learning and Memory in Rodents." **Psychopharmacology.** 1982, Vol. 78, pp. 104-11.

Foltyn, P., Lucker, P.W., Schnitker, J., Wetzelsberger, N. "A Test Model for Cerebrally-Active Drugs as Demonstrated by the Example of the New Substance Aniracetam" **Arzneimittelforschung.** 1983, 33 (6) pp. 865-7.

Gamzu, E., et al. "Pharmacological Protection Against Memory Retrieval Deficits as a Method of Discovering New Therapeutic Agents." **Alzheimer's and Parkinson's Disease: Strategies in Research and Development.** Advances in Behavioral Biology, vol. 29, New York, Plenum Press, 1986.

Pelton, R., Pelton, T.C. **Mind Food & Smart Pills.** New York: Doubleday, 1989.

Saletu, B., Grunberger, J., Linzmayer, L. "Quantitative EEG and Psychometric Analyses in Assessing CNS-Activity of RO 13-5057—a Cerebral Insufficiency Improver." **Methods and Findings in Experimental Clinical Pharmacology.** 1980, 2 (5) pp. 269-85.

Saletu, B., Grunberger, J. "The Hypoxia Model in Human Psychopharmacology: Neurophysiological and Psychometric Studies with Aniracetam I.V." **Human Neurobiology.** 1984, 3 (3) pp. 171-81.

Vincent, G., Verderese, A., Gamzu, E. "The Effects of Aniracetam (Ro-13-5057) on the Enhancement and Protection of Memory." **Annals of the New York Academy of Sciences.** 1985, Vol. 444, pp. 489-91.

Fipexide

A double-blind study involving 40 elderly people with severe cognition disorders found that fipexide improved cognition and performance on a number of different tests. One test used in the study measured several different parameters including co-ordination, short term memory and attention.

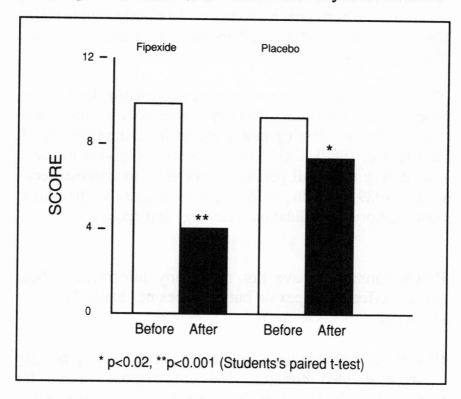

Clinical scores in patients with severe cognition disorders. The lower scores represent improvement. (Redrawn from Bompani, 1986.)

The fipexide-treated subjects reduced the time taken to complete the task by an average of 22%, and decreased their errors by 46%. The researchers calculated the average improvement in cognition at 60% (Bompani, 1986).

Fipexide has a mild dopamine-enhancing effect. Dopamine is a neurotransmitter critical to fine motor coordination, immune function, motivation and emotions. One study measured the hormonal responses of 10 elderly people taking fipexide, and found a small increase in dopamine release (Rolandi, 1984).

This smart drug may prove to be excellent for the learning process of consolidating memory. Laboratory animals given fipexide before learning new material have improved recall later (Serra, 1989). Unlike other nootropics, giving Fipexide only during the recall period did not seem to improve recall (Serra, 1989, Valzelli, 1986). Most nootropics are helpful in both memory consolidation (learning) and recall.

Precautions: We have not found any information about adverse effects of fipexide but this does not mean that there are none.

Dosage: The studies we have seen have used 600mg per day in three divided dosages. The dose-response curve for fipexide is bell-shaped as has been found for many other smart drugs.

Sources: Fipexide is not sold in the U.S. but it can be purchased by mail from the sources listed in Appendix A (see page 165). Other names include: Attentil, BP 662, Vigilor.

References:

Bompani, R., Scali G. "Fipexide, an Effective Cognition Activator in the Elderly: a Placebo-Controlled, Double-Blind Clinical Trial." **Current Medical Research and Opinion.** 1986, 10 (2) pp. 99-106.

Rolandi, E., Franceschini, R., Marabini, A., Messina, V., Bongera, P., Barreca, T. "Pituitary Secretion After Administration of a New Cerebroactive Drug, Fipexide." **British Journal of Clinical Pharmacology.** 1984, 18 (2) pp. 236-9.

Serra, G., Collu, M., Martellotta, M.C., Forgione, A., Fratta, W. "Effect of Fipexide on Passive Avoidance Behavior in Rats." **Pharmacological Research.** 1989, 21(5) pp. 603-8.

Valzelli, L., Baiguerra, G., Giraud, O. "Difference in Learning and Retention by Albino Swiss Mice. Part III. Effect of Some Brain Stimulants." **Methods and Findings in Experimental and Clinical Pharmacology.** 1986, 8(6) pp. 337-41.

Oxiracetam

Oxiracetam is another piracetam analog. One study conducted in Japan compared the effects of piracetam and oxiracetam on normal mice learning a new task called *discrete two-way shuttle avoidance*. The mice had to learn to break a photo-beam whenever they heard a warning stimulus in order to avoid a mild electric shock. The optimum dose of oxiracetam for improving learning was 30mg per kilogram of body weight, whereas the optimum dose of piracetam was 100mg per kilogram (over three times as much) (Kuribara, 1988).

An amazing study done in Italy attempted to find teratological (birth-defect causing) effects of oxiracetam. Pregnant mice were given oxiracetam from the beginning of their pregnancies until they gave birth. Controls were given saline solution instead. The offspring of the oxiracetam-treated mice showed no negative effects at birth. After one month, the offspring of oxiracetam-treated mice (remember that the offspring themselves were not being given oxiracetam) showed signs of being more curious than the offspring of the controls (Ammassari-Teule, 1988). At three months, the oxiracetam offspring were performing significantly better in memory tests than the offspring of the controls. Although this is not a recommendation for pregnant women to take oxiracetam, it certainly hints at exciting possibilities, and indicates that this is an amazing and non-toxic smart drug.

After elderly people with dementia were given oxiracetam for three months, several different tests were administered. The researchers wrote that oxiracetam is a "vigilance-enhancing compound with some effects on spontaneous memory," and that "in comparison with piracetam, oxiracetam exhibits (a) greater improvement in memory factor" (Itil, 1986).

Another oxiracetam study was performed on a large number of people. Three hundred seven people were enrolled originally and 272 people completed the study. Eight hundred milligrams of oxiracetam was given twice each day for a total of twelve weeks to patients suffering from primary degenerative, multi-infarct or mixed forms of dementia. They found significant improvements in memory and concentration (Maina, 1989).

In another study, oxiracetam and piracetam were each administered to 30 people (a total of 60 people). The dosage was a very large 6000mg per day. After 60 days of treatment, the researchers concluded that the tolerability of oxiracetam was excellent. They found that oxiracetam had better therapeutic results than piracetam on both psychosomatic and neurologic symptoms. Oxiracetam also seemed to decrease platelet aggregation (Ferrero, 1984).

Oxiracetam is currently being investigated by the SmithKline Beckman Corporation for the treatment of Alzheimer's disease. SmithKline is conducting a multi-center study of oxiracetam. There are several other companies involved with oxiracetam who see great potential for this smart drug.

Oxiracetam was originally developed by the Italian pharmaceutical company, ICF. The drug was introduced in Italy in 1988 and will probably be introduced to further European markets in 1990. ICF licensed non-European rights to Ciba-Geigy of Japan. The U.S. rights to it have recently been assigned to SmithKline Beckman Corporation. We wonder if the difficulties attendant to gaining FDA approval for nootropics is the cause of the switch. Ciba-Geigy is working with Toyo Jozo (another Japanese corporation) to get approval for sale of oxiracetam in Japan within three years. They hope for eventual world sales of $50 million (Barclays de Zoete Wedd Chemicals Research, 1987, 1988, Japan Chemical Week, 1987).

Precautions: Oxiracetam, like other nootropics, is non-toxic. It has been shown to be safe in doses up to 2400mg (Itil, 1986).

Dosage: Oxiracetam is more potent than piracetam. In one study aimed at finding the optimum dosage subjects were tested with 200mg, 400mg, 800mg, 1200mg, and 2400mg per day. The greatest improvements in cognitive function occurred at doses of 1200mg and 2400mg per day.

Sources: SmithKline hopes to soon get approval for oxiracetam in the U.S. for the treatment of Alzheimer's disease but we wouldn't hold our breath. Oxiracetam is sold in Italy. It can be purchased from the overseas sources listed in Appendix A (see page 165). Other names include: CT-848, hydroxypiracetam, ISF-2522, Neuractiv, Neuromet.

References:

Ammassari-Teule, M., D'Amato, F.R., Sansone, M., Oliverio, A. "Avoidance Facilitation in Adult Mice by Prenatal Administration of the Nootropic Drug Oxiracetam." **Pharmacological Research Communications**. 1986, Vol. 18, No. 12, pp. 1169-78

Ammassari-Teule, M., D'Amato, F.R., Sansone, M., Oliverio, A. "Enhancement of Radial Maze Performances in CD1 Mice after Prenatal Exposure to Oxiracetam: Possible Role of Sustained Investigative Responses Developed During Ontogeny." **Physiology and Behavior**. 1988, 42 (3), pp. 281-5.

Barclays de Zoete Wedd Chemicals Research. Switzerland Issue 1, June 25, 1987, pp. 4-5.

Ibid. Issue 88, July 11, 1988, pp. 5-6.

Ferrero, E. "Controlled Clinical Trial of Oxiracetam in the Treatment of Chronic Cerebrovascular Insufficiency in the Elderly." **Current Therapeutic Research**. August 1984, Vol. 36, No. 2, pp. 298-308.

Itil, T.M., Menon, G.N., Songar, A., Itil, K.Z. "CNS Pharmacology and Clinical Therapeutic Effects of Oxiracetam." **Clinical Neuropharmacology**. 1986, Vol. 9, Supplement 3. New York: Raven Press, pp. S70-S78.

Japan Chemical Week. Vol 28, Issue 1445, December 12, 1987, p. 4.

Kuribara, H., Tadokoro, S. "Facilitating Effect of Oxiracetam and Piracetam on Acquisition of Discrete Two-Way Shuttle Avoidance in Normal Mice." **Japanese Journal of Pharmacology**. 1988, 48 (4), pp. 494-8.

Maina, G., Fiori, L., Torta, R., Fagiani, M.B., Ravizza, L., Bonavita, E., Ghiazza, B., Teruzzi, F., Zagnoni, P.G., Ferrario, E., et al. "Oxiracetam in the Treatment of Primary Degenerative and Multi-Infarct Dementia: a Double-Blind, Placebo-Controlled Study." **Neuropsychobiology**. 1989, 21 (3), pp. 141-5.

Mondadori, C., Classen, W., Borkowski, J., Ducret, T., Buerki, H., Schade, A. "Effects of Oxiracetam on Learning and Memory in Animals: Comparison with Piracetam." **Clinical Neuropharmacology**. 1986, Vol. 9, Supplement 13. New York: Raven Press, pp. S27-S37.

Pramiracetam

The pharmaceutical firm of Parke Davis has developed a variation of the piracetam molecule called pramiracetam. Pramiracetam enhances the functioning of the cholinergic system in a manner similar to that of piracetam, but it is effective at much lower doses.

In one study, subjects with Alzheimer's disease showed significant intelligence and memory enhancement with only 150mg per day of pramiracetam (Poschel, 1983). Piracetam requires doses of 2.5 to 4.8 grams per day to get the same sort of responses. In other words, pramiracetam is about 15 times more powerful than piracetam.

In some research, pramiracetam has proven more effective than piracetam in the treatment of Alzheimer's disease (Branconnier, 1983). Parke Davis is spending a great deal of money to gain FDA approval for selling pramiracetam as a treatment for Alzheimer's disease.

Precautions: Preliminary findings indicate that, like other nootropics, it has little or no toxicity and no or few side effects (DeJong, 1987).

Dosage: 75-1500mg (DeJong, 1987, Itil, 1983).

Sources: As of this writing, we have not found pramiracetam for sale in the U.S. or overseas. When it does become available in other countries, U.S. doctors can legally prescribe it for whatever use they see fit. Other names include: CI-879.

References:

Branconnier, R. "The Efficacy of the Cerebral Metabolic Enhancers in the Treatment of Senile Dementia." **Psychopharmacology Bulletin.** 1983, 19(2), pp. 212-20.

Branconnier, R.J., Cole, J.O., Dessain, E.C., Spera, K.F., Ghazvinian, S., DeVitt, D. "The Therapeutic Efficacy of Pramiracetam in Alzheimer's Disease: Preliminary Observations." **Psychopharmacology Bulletin.** 1983, 19(4), pp. 726-30.

DeJong, R. "Safety of Pramiracetam." **Current Therapeutic Research.** 1987, 41(2), pp. 254-7.

Itil, T.M. **"Pramiracetam, A New Nootropic: A Controlled Quantitative Pharmaco-Electroencephalographic Study."** Psychopharmacology Bulletin. 1983, Vol. 19, No. 4, pp. 708-16.

Murray, C.L., Fibiger, H.C. "The Effect of Pramiracetam (CI-879) on the Acquisition of a Radial Arm Maze Task." **Psychopharmacology**. 1986, Vol. 89, pp. 378-81.

Pelton, R., Pelton, T.C. **Mind Food & Smart Pills.** New York: Doubleday, 1989.

Poschel, B.P.H., Marriott, J.G., Gluckman, M.I. "Pharmacology Underlying the Cognition-Activating Properties of Pramiracetam (CI-879)." **Psychopharmacology Bulletin.** 1983, Vol. 19, 4, pp. 720-1.

Pyroglutamate (PCA)

Pyroglutamate (also called 2-oxo-pyrrolidone carboxylic acid, or PCA) is an amino acid naturally occurring in vegetables, fruits, dairy products, and meat, and seems to be an important flavor constituent in these foods. It is also normally present in large amounts in the human brain, cerebrospinal fluid, and blood. Pyroglutamate is known to have a number of remarkable cognitive-enhancing effects.

After oral administration, pyroglutamate passes into the brain through the blood-brain barrier and stimulates cognitive functions. Pyroglutamate improves memory and learning in rats, and has anti-anxiety effects in rats (Pearson and Shaw, 1988).

Pyroglutamate has also been shown to be effective in alcohol-induced memory deficits in humans (Sinforiani, 1985) and, more recently, in people affected with multi-infarct dementia (Scoppa, in press). In these patients, the administration of pyroglutamate brought about a significant increase of attention and an improvement on psychological tests investigating short-term retrieval, long-term retrieval, and long-term storage of memory. A statistically significant improvement was observed also in the consolidation of memory.

In human subjects, pyroglutamate was compared with placebo in a randomized double-blind trial for assessing its

67

efficacy in treating memory deficits in 40 aged subjects. Twenty subjects were treated with pyroglutamate and 20 with placebo over a period of 60 days. Memory functions were evaluated at baseline and after 60 days of treatment by means of a battery made up of six memory tasks. The results show that pyroglutamate is effective in improving verbal memory functions in subjects affected by age-related memory decline (Grioli, 1990).

In Italy, arginine pyroglutamate (one source of pyro-glutamate) is used to treat senility, mental retardation, and alcoholism (Anderson, 1987). Arginine pyroglutamate is simply an arginine molecule combined with a pyroglutamate molecule. Arginine alone does not produce cognitive enhanc-ing effects. It is likely that pyroglutamate is the active ingredient of arginine pyroglutamate.

Some people use arginine, a single amino acid, to build muscle bulk and to burn fat because the arginine causes the pituitary gland to release natural growth hormone. Arginine pyroglutamate, in addition to having cognitive enhancing effects, is an excellent growth hormone releaser because it is carried more efficiently across the blood-brain barrier than arginine alone (Filipo, 1987).

Many people have told us that they like the effects of arginine pyroglutamate a great deal. Some of the more interesting anecdotes are listed in Appendix D (see page 179).

Precautions: No serious adverse effects from the use of pyroglutamate, or from the use of arginine pyroglutamate, have been reported. Arginine and pyroglutamate are amino acids found commonly in natural foods and consumed by most people on a regular basis.

Dosage: 500mg to 1000mg per day for arginine pyroglutamate or somewhat less if straight pyroglutamate is used.

Sources: Health food and vitamin stores offer various products containing pyroglutamate, including Amino Mass and Mental Edge from Source Naturals, and Deep Thought from KAL. Arginine pyroglutamate (one source of pyroglutamate) is often used for its growth-hormone releasing effect, but is still effective as a cognitive enhancer in this form. Other names for pyroglutamate include: alpha-aminoglutaric acid lactam, glutamic acid lactam, glutimic acid, glutiminic acid, pyroGlu, and pyroglutamic acid. Other names for arginine pyroglutamate include: Adjuvant, Piraglutargine, Arginine Pidolate.

References:

Anderson, K., Anderson, L. **Orphan Drugs**. Los Angeles, CA: The Body Press, 1987, p. 170.

Cenni, A., et al. "Pharmacological Properties of a Nootropic Agent of Endogenous Origin: D-Pyroglutamic Acid." **Journal of Drug Development**. 1988, 1, pp. 157-62.

Chemical Business. September 1988, p. 43.

Drago, F., Continella, G., Valerio, C., D'Agata, V., Astuto, C., Spardaro, F., Scapagnini, U. "Effects of Pyroglutamic Acid on Learning and Memory Processes of the Rat." **Acta Therapeutica**. 1987, Vol. 13, pp. 587-94.

Filippo, V., Spignoli, G., Isidori, A. "Effects of Arginine Pyroglutamate on Growth Hormone in Children." **Clinical Trials Journal**. 1987, Vol. 24, pp. 387-90.

Grioli, S. et al. "Pyroglutamic Acid Improves the Age Associated Memory Impairment." **Fundamental and Clinical Pharmacolo-**

gy. 1990, Vol. 4, pp. 169-73.

Moret, C., Briley, M. "The Forgotten Amino Acid Pyroglutamate." **Trends in Pharmacological Sciences.** 1988, Vol. 9, pp. 278-9.

Paoli, F., Spignoli, G., Pepeu, G. "Oxiracetam and D-Pyroglutamic Acid Antagonize a Disruption of Passive Avoidance Behavior Induced by the N-Methyl-Aspartate Receptor Antagonist 2-amino-5-phosphonovalerate." **Psychopharmacology.** 1990, 100, pp. 130-1.

Pearson, D., Shaw, S. **Durk Pearson & Sandy Shaw's Life Extension Newsletter.** October 1988, Vol 1, Number 8, p. 65-66.

Pepeu, G., Spignoli, G. "Neurochemical Actions of Nootropic Drugs". **Advances in Neurology. Vol. 51: Alzheimer's Disease.** New York: Raven Press, Ltd., 1990.

Porsolt, R.D., Lenegre, A., Avril, I., Parot, P., Tran, G. "Antiamnesic Effects of Magnesium Pyrrolidone Carboxylate (MAG 2) in Three Models of Amnesia in the Mouse." **Drug Development Research.** 1988, 13, pp. 57-67.

Sinforiani, E., Trucco, M., Cavallini, A., Gualtieri, S., Verri, A.P., Spignoli, G. "Sulla Reversibilita Dei Disordini Cognitivi Negli Alcolisti Cronici In Fase Di Dissauefazion." **Minerva Psichiatrica.** 1985, 26, pp. 339-42.

Spignoli, G., Magnani, M. Pepeu, G. "Pyroglutamic Acid Antagonizes the Amnesic Effect and the Decrease in Brain Acetylcholine Level Induced by Scopolamine." **Pharmacological Research Communications.** 1987, Vol. 10, pp. 901-7.

Vinpocetine (Cavinton)

Vinpocetine is a powerful memory enhancer. It facilitates cerebral metabolism by improving cerebral microcirculation (blood flow), stepping up brain cell ATP production (ATP is the cellular energy molecule), and increasing utilization of glucose and oxygen.

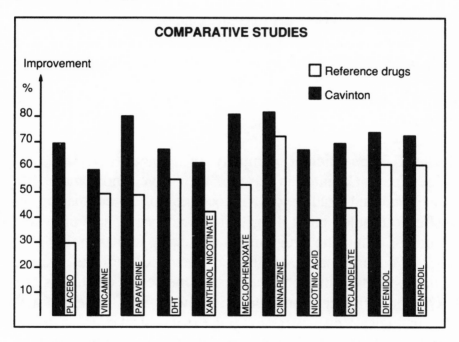

This graph represents comparative studies of vinpocetine and other smart drugs. (Redrawn from Gedeon Richter, Ltd. product literature.)

What all this means is that vinpocetine shares many of the effects of several other cognitive enhancers. In the above graph from a piece of drug company literature, vinpocetine is shown to compare favorably to: placebo, vincamine, papaverine, DHT (Hydergine), xanthinol nicotinate, meclophenoxate, cinnarizine, niacin, cyclandelate, difenidol, and ifenprodil.

Vinpocetine is often used for the treatment of cerebral circulatory disorders such as memory problems, acute stroke, aphasia (loss of the power of expression), apraxia (inability to coordinate movements), motor disorders, dizziness and other cerebro-vestibular (inner-ear) problems, and headache. Vinpocetine is also used to treat acute or chronic ophthalmological diseases of various origin, with visual acuity improving in 70% of the subjects.

Vinpocetine also is used in the treatment of sensorineural hearing impairment.

The Gedeon Richter company of Hungary markets vinpocetine as Cavinton in Europe. They have funded more than one hundred studies on vinpocetine, often comparing its effects to other smart drugs. The incidence of side effects in humans using the drug orally is usually less than 1% of a study's participants, with the unwanted effects usually disappearing with continued use. One series of studies that Gedeon Richter conducted involved 882 patients with neurological disorders ranging from stroke to cerebral insufficiency. Significant improvements were found in 62% of the patients. In one of the studies, cerebral insufficiency patients were asked to memorize a list of 10 words. Without vinpocetine the subjects were able to memorize an average of 6 words. After a month of treatment the average went up to 10 words. Gedeon Richter promotes vinpocetine as the only drug that improves cerebral metabolism (glucose and oxygen uptake), tolerance of hypoxia (deficient blood oxygenation), ATP concentration, norepinephrine and serotonin turnover, and cerebral microcirculation. Gedeon Richter also claims that vinpocetine selectively increases blood flow to the brain, improving blood flow to the impaired area without lowering blood flow to other parts of the body (Gedeon Richter product literature).

Vincamine

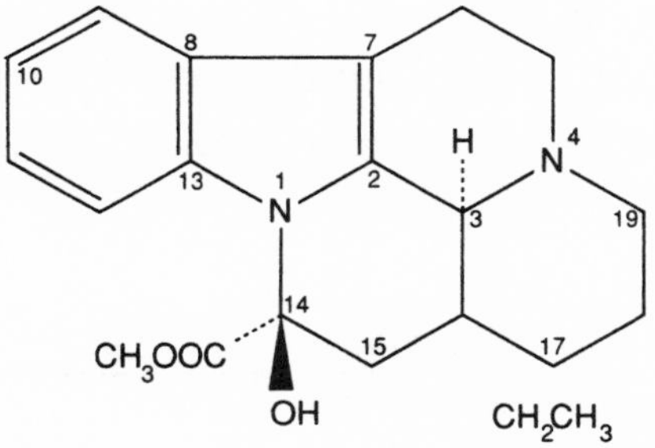

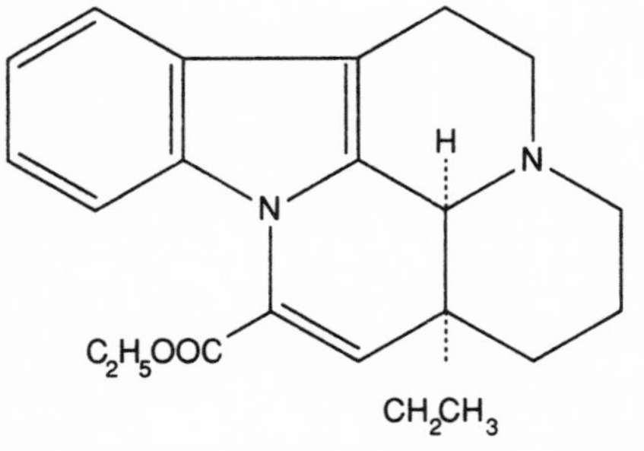

Vinpocetine

As if the medical uses of vinpocetine were not amazing enough, in one double-blind crossover study normal, healthy volunteers showed incredible short-term memory improvement an hour after taking 40mg of vinpocetine. The volunteers took a computer-administered short-term memory test called a Sternberg Memory Scanning Test. The volunteers (all women between the ages of 25 and 40) were shown one to three digits on a computer screen, then a moment later were shown a long string of digits. The volunteers then indicated whether any of the first digits appeared in the second long string. The time the volunteer took to remember was then assessed. On a placebo the women took an average of 700 milliseconds to respond when the first set contained 3 digits. With vinpocetine they averaged under 450 milliseconds! (Subhan, 1985).

Vinpocetine is a derivative of vincamine, which is an extract of the periwinkle. Although they have many similar effects vinpocetine has more benefits and fewer adverse effects than vincamine.

Symptoms	Improved, %
Dizziness	**77.1**
Headache	**77.7**
Numbness	**70.8**
Depressed mood	**73.6**
Irritability	**73.4**
Mood instability	**66.4**
Insomnia	**70.3**
Instable blood pressure	**86.9**
Ataxia	**64.6**
Paretic symptoms	**57.8**
Aphasia	**60.0**
Speech disturbances	**55.7**
Attention, concentration disorders	**65.3**
Memory disturbances	**62.3**
Slow thinking	**56.1**
Nervousness	**82.7**

Percentage of patients taking vinpocetine whose symptoms of cerebrovascular disorders improved. (Redrawn from Gedeon Richter, Ltd. product literature.)

Precautions: Adverse effects are rare, but include hypotension, dry mouth, weakness, and tachycardia. Vinpocetine has no known drug interactions, no toxicity, and is generally very safe.

Dosage: One or two 5 mg tablets per day.

Sources: Vinpocetine is not sold in the U.S. It can be purchased by mail order from the sources listed in Appendix A (see page 165). Other names include: ARGH-4405, Cavinton, Ceractin.

References:

DeNoble, V.J., Repetti, S.J., Gelpke, L.W., Wood, L.M., Keim, K.L. "Vinpocetine: Nootropic Effects on Scopolamine-Induced and Hypoxia-Induced Retrieval Deficits of a Step-Through Passive Avoidance Response in Rats." **Pharmacology Biochemistry & Behavior**. 1986, Vol. 24, pp. 1123-8.

Gedeon Richter product literature, **Cavinton**.

Hadjiev, D., Yancheva, S. "Rheoencephalographic and Psychologic Studies with Ethyl Apovincaminate in Cerebral Vascular Insufficiency." **Arzneimittelforschung**. 1976, Vol. 26, pp. 1947-50.

Otomo, E., Atarashi, J., Araki, G., Ito, E., Omae, T., Kuzuya, F., Nukada, T., Ebi, O. "Comparison of Vinpocetine with Ifenprodil Tartrate and Dihydroergotoxine Mesylate Treatment and Results of Long-Term Treatment with Vinpocetine." **Current Therapeutic Research**. 1985, Vol. 37, No. 5, pp. 811-21.

Pelton, R., Pelton, T.C. **Mind Food & Smart Pills**. New York: Doubleday, 1989.

Subhan, Z., Hindmarch, I. "Psychopharmacological Effects of Vinpocetine in Normal Healthy Volunteers." **European Journal of Clinical Pharmacology**. 1985, Vol. 28, pp. 567-71.

Other Cognitive Enhancers

Acetyl-L-Carnitine (ALC)

This naturally-occurring molecule is involved in the transport of fats into the mitochondria, the energy-producing part of all living cells, and is found in some common foods such as milk. Acetyl-L-carnitine is related to choline compounds, both chemically and in clinical effects.

In animal studies, long-term administration of ALC preserves spatial memory in aged rats (Ghirardi, 1989), and improved learning and memory in mice and rats (Bossoni, 1986, Drago, 1986).

ALC may also have some important properties of protecting the brain from the effects of aging. NMDA-sensitive glutamate receptors in the brain are important for learning, but they decrease with age. One study of these receptors in rat brains found that ALC has a neuroprotective and neurotrophic (brain-cell nourishing) effect during aging.

Of great interest to researchers is ALC's ability to inhibit the formation of lipofuscin in the brains of aged laboratory animals (Kohjimoto, 1988). The buildup of these fatty deposits in the nerve cells is associated with a reduction of cognitive powers.

In human studies, ALC has increased attention span and alertness in people with Alzheimer's disease and other forms of senility. One study using 2000mg of ALC per day showed small but significant improvements in short-term memory in people with Alzheimer's disease (Rai, 1990). Another recent study, reported at the 14th International Congress of Gerontology, found that ALC increased brain levels of choline acetyltransferase. Low levels of this enzyme are found in Alzheimer's patients, and is the major reason for their severe deficiency of acetylcholine (Pearson and Shaw, 1990).

One study treated 20 patients with 1500mg ALC per day for six months. All patients had involutional symptoms (the regressive changes in the body occurring with old age). They were being treated by a rehabilitation therapist for their concomitant decrease of motor activities. This long term study found that the patients improved on measures of cognitive ability, depression, and self-sufficiency. It also found an improvement in social life and motor activity in these patients (Fiore, 1989).

Another study gave 500mg of ALC per day to a group of 20 persons with senility (20 others were given placebo). The researchers found a significant improvement in several measures of senility (Bonavita, 1986).

In one study of hospitalized geriatric patients, ALC was shown to be effective for the treatment of depression (Tempesta, 1987).

Precautions: Studies on humans have not found any toxic effects or significant side effects (Bonavita, 1986, Tempesta, 1987). This does not mean that there are no negative effects. It only means we have not seen any evidence for negative effects.

Dosage: 1000mg-2000mg per day in two divided doses.

Sources: We know of no source in the U.S. for ALC, although since it is a naturally-occurring substance it could be legally sold in health food stores (Snoswell, 1975). Therefore, we would expect health-food-industry distributors to add this compound to their product line very shortly after they find out about it from this book. ALC is available in Europe and by mail order from the sources listed in Appendix A (see page 165). Other names for ALC include: Alcar, Branigen, levacecarnine hydrochloride, n-acetyl-l-carnitine, Nicetile, and ST-200.

References:

Albano, C. "Evaluation of the Activity of Acetyl-L-Carnitine in the Senile Dementia Alzheimer Type." **Abstract of IVth World Congress of Biological Psychiatry**, Philadelphia, 1985, p. 106.

Bonavita, E. "Study of the Efficacy and Tolerability of L-Acetylcarnitine Therapy in the Senile Brain." **Journal of Clinical Pharmacology, Therapy, and Toxicology.** 1986, 24, pp. 511-6.

Bossoni, G., Carpi C. "Effect of Acetyl-L-Carnitine on Conditioned Reflex Learning Rate and Retention in Laboratory Animals." **Drugs Under Experimental and Clinical Research.** 1986, 12 (11) pp. 911-6.

Cucinotta, D., Ventura, S., Passeri, M., Iannuccelli, M. Orfalian, Z., Senin, V., Parnetti, L., Bonati, P.A. "Clinical Experience with Acetyl-L-Carnitine in the Treatment of Signs and Symptoms of Senile Mental Deterioration in the Aged." **5th Capo Boi Conference on Neuroscience.** 1987 (Abstract).

Drago, F., Continella, G., Pennisi, G., Alloro, M.C., Calvani, M., Scapagnini, U. "Behavioral Effects of Acetyl-L-Carnitine in the Male Rat." **Pharmacology, Biochemistry, and Behavior.** 1986, 24 (5) pp. 1393-6.

Fiore, L., Rampello, L. "L-acetylcarnitine Attenuates the Age-Dependent Decrease of NMDA-Sensitive Glutamate Receptors in Rat

Hippocampus." **Acta Neurologica**. 1989, 11 (5), pp. 346-50.

Guarnaschelli, C., Fugazza, G., Pistarini, C. "Pathological Brain Aging: Evaluation of the Efficacy of a Pharmacological Aid." **Drugs Under Experimental Clinical Research**. 1988, 14 (11) pp. 715-8.

Ghirardi, O., Milano, S., Ramacci, M.T., Angelucci, L. "Long-Term Acetyl-L-Carnitine Preserves Spatial Learning in the Senescent Rat." **Progress in Neuro-psychopharmacology & Biological Psychiatry**. 1989, 13 (1-2) pp. 237-45.

Kohjimoto, Y., Ogawa, T., Matsumoto, M., Shirakawa, K., Kuwaki, T., Yasuda, H., Anami, K., Fujii, T., Satoh, H., Ono, T. "Effects of Acetyl-L-Carnitine on the Brain Lipofuscin Content and Emotional Behavior in Aged Rats." **Japanese Journal of Pharmacology**. 1988, Vol. 48, pp. 365-71.

Pearson, D., Shaw, S. **Durk Pearson & Sandy Shaw's Life Extension Newsletter**. January-February 1990, Vol 2, Number 10, pp. 84-6.

Rai, G., Wright, G., Scott, L., Beston, B., Rest, J., Exton-Smith, A.N. "Double-Blind, Placebo Controlled Study of Acetyl-L-Carnitine in Patients with Alzheimer's Dementia." **Current Medical Research and Opinion**. 1990, 11 (10) pp. 638-47.

Snoswell, A.M., Linzell, J.L. "Carnitine Secretion Into Milk of Ruminants." Department of Agricultural Biochemistry, Waite Agricultural Research Institute, University of Adelaide, Glen Osmond, S. Australia 5064, Australia.

Tempesta, E., Casella, L., Pirrongelli, C., Janiri, L., Calvani, M., Ancona, L. "L-acetylcarnitine in Depressed Elderly Subjects. A Cross-Over Study vs. Placebo." **Drugs Under Experimental Clinical Research**. 1987, 13 (7) pp. 417-23.

Caffeine

Caffeine is widely used for its stimulant properties. Most people think of caffeine as improving their ability to think clearly, but a great deal of the research shows that it actually does not improve human memory in a variety of psychological tests.

One study administered 100mg doses of caffeine to normal, healthy college students and found that their ability to remember lists of words that they had just heard was diminished when they were given caffeine (Terry, 1986). In another study, college students were given either 0, 2, or 4mg of caffeine for every kilogram of their body weight. At the 2mg rate, that would be 127mg for a 140 lb. person. A 5 oz. cup of coffee can contain from 40 - 180 mg caffeine. Female students had a more difficult time of remembering lists of words that were read to them slowly when they were given caffeine, and otherwise no memory effects, good or bad were noted by the researchers (Erikson, 1985). Thirty-two normal, healthy men were randomly given 0, 125, 250mg of caffeine and then given a recall test, a reaction time test, and a Stroop color word test that involves confusing data. They performed poorly with the high dose on the Stroop test. The researchers wrote, "Caffeine may have a deleterious effect on the rapid processing of ambiguous or confusing stimuli..." (Foreman, 1989). This sounds like a description of modern life.

A 1983 study found that combining caffeine and alcohol actually slowed the reaction time of 8 subjects. The caffeine and alcohol combination made the subjects more drunk than alcohol alone (Oborne, 1983). So much for the popular myth that giving a drunk some coffee is a good way to get him or her back on the road.

Coffee contains many chemicals other than caffeine. There are at least three opiate-like compounds in coffee. This probably accounts for coffee drinkers describing coffee as relaxing. These opiate-like compounds, which are found even in decaffeinated coffee, may also in part account for coffee's addictive qualities.

People desiring a mild, non-toxic stimulant that improves memory and cognitive functions should consider the nootropics, described earlier in this book.

References:

Baer, R. "Effects of Caffeine on Classroom Behavior, Sustained Attention, and a Memory Task in Preschool Children." **Journal of Applied Behavior Analysis**. 1987, 20 (3) pp. 225-34.

Erikson, G.C., Hager, L.B., Houseworth, C., Dungan, J., Petros, T., Beckwith, B.E. "The Effects of Caffeine on Memory for Word Lists." **Physiology and Behavior**. 1985, 35 (1), pp. 47-51.

Foreman, N., Barraclough, S., Moore, C., Mehta, A., Madon, M. "High Doses of Caffeine Impair Performance of a Numerical Version of the Stroop Task in Men." **Pharmacology, Biochemistry, and Behavior**. 1989, 32 (2) pp. 399-403.

Oborne, D., Rogers, Y. "Interactions of Alcohol and Caffeine on Human Reaction Time." **Aviation, Space, and Environmental Medicine**. 1983, 54 (6) pp. 528-34.

Terry, W., Phifer, B. "Caffeine and Memory Performance on the AVLT." **Journal of Clinical Psychology**. 1986, 42 (6) p.860.

Centrophenoxine (Lucidril)

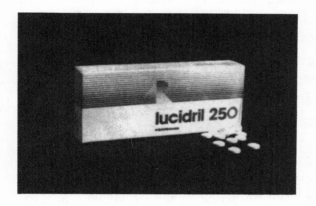

Centrophenoxine is an intelligence booster and may also be an effective anti-aging therapy. It has been shown to cause improvements in various aspects of memory function and a 30% increase in life span of laboratory animals (Hochschild, 1973).

One of the most widely recognized aspects of aging is the build-up of lipofuscin in brain cells, heart, and skin (lipofuscin is the stuff of which "age spots" are made). In animal studies, decreased lipofuscin deposits have been correlated with improved learning ability, and, conversely, increased lipofuscin deposits have been correlated with decreased learning ability (Nandy, 1988).

Centrophenoxine removes lipofuscin deposits (Nandy, 1966, 1978). It also repairs the synapses, which is where the neurotransmitters are released from one nerve cell in order to convey information to another.

Centrophenoxine breaks down into DMAE (see page 99) in the blood stream. Some researchers have suggested that centrophenoxine's effects may be identical to DMAE's. One study found that DMAE and Centrophenoxine had the same free-radical-scavenging abilities (Nagy, 1984). However, another piece of research indicates that Centrophenoxine is better than DMAE in retarding lipofuscin accumulation in a nematode (Zuckerman, 1978).

Centrophenoxine has been shown to protect the brains of animals from hypoxia (lack of oxygen) (Miyazaki, 1976). It may be of value in treating some cases of stroke, athero-sclerotic dementia, angina, intermittent claudication, and other conditions in which oxygenation of tissues is reduced (Dowson, 1988).

Centrophenoxine is probably not effective in treating Alz-heimer's disease (Branconnier, 1983). However, some research indicates it may be useful in cases where hypoxia is speeding the development of the disease (Gedye, 1972; Mercer, 1972). Centrophenoxine should be begun in the early stages of Alzheimer's disease (Dowson, 1988).

Precautions: Centrophenoxine should not be used by persons who are easily excitable, have severe hypertension, or are subject to convulsions or involuntary musculoskeletal move-ments. Centrophenoxine also should not be used by nursing mothers. Adverse effects are rare, but include hyperexcitabil-ity, insomnia, tremors, motion sickness, paradoxical drowsi-ness and depression. If taken late in the day, centrophenoxine is more likely to cause insomnia. There is no toxicity of centrophenoxine at therapeutic doses.

Dosage: 1000 to 3000 mg per day. Centrophenoxine takes effect very quickly. Many people notice an increase in alertness and a slight stimulation effect.

Sources: Centrophenoxine is not sold in the U.S. It can be purchased over the counter in Mexico or by mail order from the sources listed in Appendix A (see page 165). Other names include: acephen, Analux, ANP 235, Brenal, Cellative, Cerebon, Cerebron, Cetrexin, Clocete, clofenoxine, Helfergin, Licidril, Lucidril, Luncidril, Lutiaron, Marucotol, meclofenoxane, meclofenoxate, Mecloxate, Methoxynal, Proserout, Proseryl, Ropoxyl, and Telucidone.

References:

Anderson, K., Anderson, L. **Orphan Drugs**. Los Angeles, CA: The Body Press, 1987, p. 132.

Dowson, J.H., Wilton-Cox, H. "The Effect of Drugs on Neuronal Lipopigment" **Lipofuscin—1987: State of the Art**. Nagy (ed), Amsterdam: Elsevier Science Publishers, 1988, pp. 271-88.

Gedye, J.L., Exton-Smith, A.N., Wedgewood, J. "A Method for Measuring Mental Performance in the Elderly and its Use in a Pilot Clinical Trial of Meclofenoxate in Organic Dementia." **Age and Ageing**. 1972, 1, pp. 74-80.

Hochschild, R. "Effect of Dimethylaminoethyl p-Chlorophenoxy-acetate on the Life Span of Male Swiss Webster Albino Mice." **Experimental Gerontology**. 1973, Vol. 8, pp. 177-83.

Jarvik, L.F. "The Aging Nervous System: Clinical Aspects." **Aging**. New York: Raven Press, 1975, Vol. 1, pp. 1-9.

Marcer, D., Hopkins, S.M. "The Differential Effects of Meclofenoxate on Memory Loss in the Elderly." **Age and Ageing**. 1977, Vol. 6, pp. 123-31.

Miyazki, H., Nambu, K., Hashimoto, M. "Antianoxic Effect of Meclofenoxate Related to its Disposition." **Chemical Pharmaceutical**

Bulletin. 1976, 24: pp. 822-25.

Nagy, I., Floyd, R. "Electron Spin Resonance Spectroscopic Demonstration of the Hydroxyl Free Radical Scavenger Properties of Dimethylaminoethanol in Spin Trapping Experiments Confirming the Molecular Basis for the Biological Effects of Centrophenoxine." **Archives of Gerontology and Geriatrics**. 1984, 3 (4) pp. 297-310.

Nandy, K. "Aging Neurons and Pharmacological Agents." **Aging**. New York: Raven Press, 1983, Vol. 21, pp. 401-15.

Nandy, K. "Lipofuscinogenesis in Mice Early Treated with Centrophenoxine." **Mechanisms of Aging and Development**. 1978, Vol. 8, pp. 131-8.

Nandy, K., Bourne, G.H. "Effect of Centrophenoxine on the Lipofuscin Pigments of the Neurones of Senile Guinea Pigs." **Nature**. 1966, Vol. 210, pp. 313-4.

Nandy, K., Mostofsky, D.I., Idrobo, F., Blatt, L., Nandy, S. "Experimental Manipulations of Lipofuscin Formation in Aging Mammals." **Lipofuscin—1987: State of the Art**. Nagy, I. (ed), Amsterdam: Elsevier Science Publishers, 1988, pp. 289-304.

Pearson, D., Shaw, S. **Life Extension: A Practical Scientific Approach**. New York: Warner Books, 1982.

Pelton, R., Pelton, T.C. **Mind Food & Smart Pills**. New York: Doubleday, 1989.

Riga, S., Riga, D. "Effects of Centrophenoxine on the Lipofuscin Pigments of the Nervous System of Old Rats." **Brain Research**. 1974, Vol. 72, pp. 265-75.

Zuckerman, B., Barrett, K. "Effects of PCA and DMAE on the Nematode Caenorhabditis Briggsae." **Experimental Aging Research**. 1978, 4 (2) pp. 133-9.

Choline & Lecithin

Choline is the precursor of acetylcholine (a neurotransmitter that plays an important role in memory). Choline improves memory by increasing the amount of acetylcholine in the brain.

Choline can be found in health food and vitamin stores in several forms including choline bitartrate, choline chloride, and phosphatidyl choline. Phosphatidyl choline (PC) is the active ingredient of lecithin.

Choline, in its various forms, has been shown to improve performance by normal, healthy humans in a variety of intelligence and memory tests (Sitaram, 1978).

PC has some unique effects as well. PC is a source of the materials from which every cell membrane in your body is made. Since most of the important electro-chemical activities in the cell arise from the membranes, PC is very important. Nerve and brain cells in particular need large quantities of PC for repair and maintenance. It also aids in the metabolism of fats, regulates blood cholesterol, and nourishes the fat-like sheaths of nerve fibers.

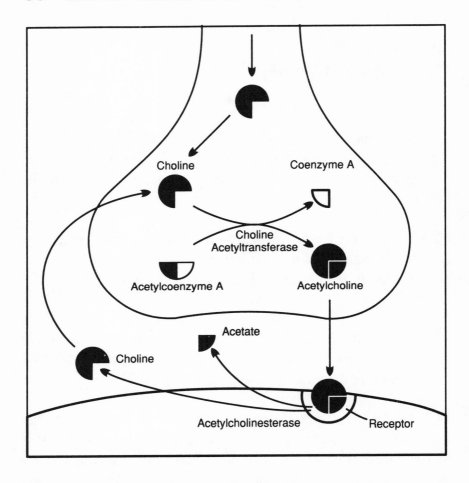

Recycling of choline at the synapse, the site of communication between nerve cells. Many cognition-enhancement compounds, including choline, work by increasing available acetylcholine at the synapse. (Redrawn from Hospital Practice, 1978.)

Precautions: Any compound that acts as a precursor to acetylcholine such as choline, PC, or DMAE should not be used by people who are manic depressive because it can deepen the depressive phase. Choline bitartrate and choline chloride can sometimes cause a fishy odor or diarrhea. PC, however, does not have either of these effects.

Dosage: 3 grams of choline per day in three divided doses. If lecithin is used as a source of choline, you may want to take more than the 3 grams, because only part of the lecithin is choline. Often the label will provide information on the quantity of choline per tablespoon. All forms of choline should be taken with one gram per day of vitamin B-5 so that the choline can be converted into acetylcholine.

Sources: Choline and lecithin are nutritional supplements that can be found at health food or drug stores. Commercial lecithin usually contains other oils and phosphatides besides phosphatidyl choline. Look at the label before you buy, and make sure the product contains more than 30% phosphatidyl choline. Lecithin easily becomes rancid, and there is no way to guarantee that the lecithin you buy is fresh. The best way is to buy your lecithin from a high-volume health food store which has a high product turnover. A high quality lecithin will have a pleasant, slightly sweet taste. TwinLab sells a product called PC-55 which is an excellent soy lecithin product. Durk Pearson and Sandy Shaw have designed a good tasting drink mix that contains choline and all of the co-factors necessary for the brain to manufacture acetylcholine. Appendix A on page 165 lists sources for these products.

References:

Gelenberg, A., et al. "Lecithin for the Treatment of Tardive Dyskine-sia." **Nutrition and the Brain.** 1979, Vol. 5, pp. 285-90.

Pearson, D., Shaw, S. **Life Extension: A Practical Scientific Approach.** New York: Warner Books, 1982.

Pelton, R., Pelton, T.C. **Mind Food & Smart Pills.** New York: Doubleday, 1989.

Sitaram, N., Weingartner, H. "Human Serial Learning: Enhancement with Arecoline and Choline and Impairment with Scopolamine." **Science.** 1978, 201, pp. 275-76.

Werbach, M. **Nutritional Influences on Illness.** Tarzana, CA: Third Line Press, 1988.

AL721 (Egg Lecithin)

AL721 is the name given to a particular extract of egg yolk by Israeli researchers. The 721 refers to 7 parts neutral lipids (oil), 2 parts phosphatidyl choline, and 1 part phosphatidyl ethanolamine.

AL721 has been used to treat senility and viral diseases such as AIDS in Israel. Several theories have been formulated to explain its action. The researchers who developed AL721 suggest that the substance increases the "fluidity" of cell membranes. They were looking for a fluidizing substance after discovering that cell membranes in aged animals were more stiff than in young animals. Since most of the electro-chemical activity in the cell originates on membranes, the fluidizing effect of AL721 could be stabilizing and "de-aging" the cell's metabolism.

Others in the field have suggested that AL721 works similar-ly to soy lecithin, improving intelligence and immune response by providing the raw materials needed by the cell to manufacture and repair the membranes. Still others call AL721 merely an expensive source of acetylcholine precur-sors.

Whether these theories are true or not, people with AIDS began to demand AL721 after preliminary research by the Israeli team suggested that it might alleviate some of the symptoms of AIDS. The researchers also gave AL721 to a number of elderly people (reportedly including at least one researcher's mother). These people were supposed to have reported improved cognition with AL721. When AL721 became available in health food stores, many people similarly began to report improved cognitive abilities with its use. Of course, this evidence is anecdotal but these reports agree with the many experiments using soy phosphatidyl choline to improve human cognition.

Precautions: Any compound that acts as a precursor to acetylcholine should not be used by people who are manic depressive because it can deepen the depressive phase.

Dosage: Like soy PC, AL721 is very safe. People with AIDS have used as much as 30 to 40 GRAMS a day of AL721. For cognitive enhancement, 2 to 10 grams per day is probably the correct dose. All forms of choline should be taken with one gram per day of vitamin B-5 so that the choline can be converted into acetylcholine.

Sources: AL721 is available under the name EggsACT from health food stores and some companies listed in Appendix A (see page 165).

References:

Shinitzky, M., et al. "Intervention in Membrane Aging - the Develop-
      ment and Application of Active Lipid." **Intervention in the
      Aging Process: Basic Research and Preclinical Screening.**
      New York: Alan R. Liss, 1983.
Shinitzky, M. (ed) **Physiology of Membrane Fluidity,** Vols. 1 & 2,
      Boca Raton, FL: CRC Press, 1984.

DHEA

DHEA or dehydroepiandrosterone (pronounced dee-hi-dro-epp-ee-an-dro-ster-own) is a steroid hormone produced in the adrenal gland. DHEA is the most abundant steroid in the human bloodstream. Research has found it to have significant anti-obesity, anti-tumor, anti-aging, and anti-cancer effects. DHEA levels naturally drop as people age, and there is good reason to think that taking a DHEA supplement may extend your life and make you more youthful while you're alive. Additionally, DHEA may be an important player in cognitive enhancement.

DHEA protects brain cells from Alzheimer's disease and other senility-associated degenerative conditions. Nerve degeneration occurs most readily under low DHEA conditions. Brain tissue naturally contains 6.5 times more DHEA than is found in the bloodstream in order to protect the brain from aging damage. Dr. Eugene Roberts found that by adding low concentrations of DHEA to nerve cell tissue cultures he could "increase the number of neurons, their ability to establish contacts, and their differentiation." DHEA also enhances long-term memory in mice. Perhaps it plays a similar role in human brain function (Fowkes, 1988; The Independent, 1989).

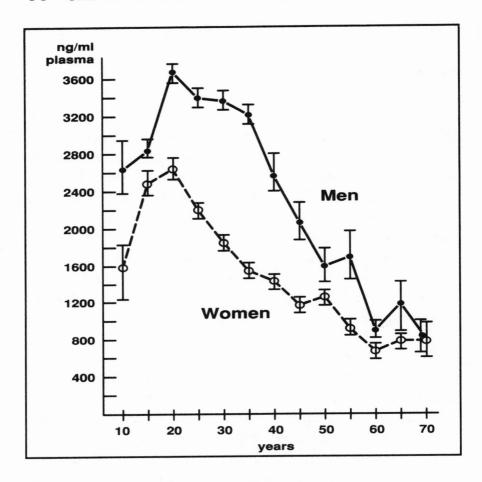

Changes in serum DHEA-S (DHEA Sulfate) levels with age. (Redrawn from Finch and Mobbs, 1982)

DHEA is now being administered to Alzheimer's patients in scientific studies. People with Alzheimer's disease have 48% less DHEA than matched controls of the same age (The Independent, 1989).

We don't know what to conclude from this result. Maybe Alzheimer's disease causes low DHEA levels or maybe vice versa. We would like to see somebody follow a large group of people over time and see if people with low DHEA levels are more likely to develop Alzheimer's disease later in life.

Precautions: DHEA use is experimental. Very little is known about long-term human use. Some women who have tried DHEA report slight increases in facial hair.

Dosage: DHEA is used in ranges of from 50 to 2000mg per day. There is no solid information indicating optimal dosage for humans, but if you want to get serious, you can get your DHEA levels tested every few months (for about $65), each time adjusting the amount of DHEA you take. Stop increasing the dose when your blood levels reach that of a 20 year old human. DHEA has a dose-dependent inverted U curve typical for smart drugs (Flood, 1988).

Sources: DHEA is now being used by many people with AIDS because of its immune-enhancing and antiviral effects. Non-profit buyer's clubs make DHEA available in the U.S. for people with AIDS. Try contacting the buyer's clubs listed in Appendix A (see page 165). The overseas sources listed in Appendix A also offer DHEA. Other names include: Astenile, Deandros, dehydroepiandrosterone, dehydroisoandrosterone, Diandron, Prasterone, Psicosterone, and trans-dehydroandrosterone.

References:

Bologa L., Sharma, J., Roberts, E. "Dehydroepiandrosterone and It's Sulfated Derivative Reduce Neuronal Death and Enhance Astrocytic Differentiation in Brain Cell Cultures." **Journal of Neuroscience Research.** 1987, 17 (3) pp. 225-34.

Cleary, M., Zisk, J. "Anti-Obesity Effect of Two Different Levels of
Dehydroepiandrosterone in Lean and Obese Middle-Aged Zucker
Rats." International Journal of Obesity. 1986, 10(3), pp.
193-204.

Dean, W. Biological Aging Measurement: Clinical Applications. Los
Angeles: Center for Bio-Gerontology, 1988.

Finch, C.E., Mobbs, C.V. "Biological Measurements Involving Steroids
and Neurotransmitters as Reflections of Physiological Aging."
Biological Markers of Aging. 1982, pp. 30-41.

Flood, J.F., Roberts, E. "Dehydroepiandrosterone Sulfate Improves
Memory in Aging Mice." Brain Research. 1988, 448 (1) pp.
178-81.

Flood, J.F., Roberts, E. "Dehydroepiandrosterone and its Sulfate
Enhance Memory Retention in Mice." Brain Research. 1988,
447 (2), pp. 269-78.

Fowkes, S. Journal of the MegaHealth Society. May, 1988, Vol. 4,
number 3, issue 17, pp. 6-7.

The Independent September 1, 1989, pp. 6.

Mohan, P.F. "Dehydroepiandrosterone and Alzheimer's Disease." [letter]
Lancet. 1989, 2 (8670) pp. 1048-9.

Pearson, D., Shaw, S. Life Extension: A Practical Scientific Approach. New York: Warner Books, 1982.

Roberts, E., Bologa, L., Flood, J.F., Smith, G.E. "Effects of Dehydroepiandrosterone and Its Sulfate on Brain Tissue in Culture and
on Memory in Mice." Brain Research. 1987, 406 (1-2) pp.
357-62.

Sunderland, T., Merril, C.R., Harrington, M.G., Lawlor, B.A.,
Molchan, S.E., Martinez, R., Murphy, D.L. "Reduced Plasma
Dehydroepiandrosterone Concentrations in Alzheimer's Dis-
ease." [letter] Lancet. 1989, 2 (8662) pp. 570.

Svec, F., Lopez, A. "Antiglucocorticoid Actions of Dehydroepiandrosterone and Low Concentrations in Alzheimer's Disease."
[letter] Lancet. 1989, 2 (8675) pp. 1335-6.

Weindruch, R., et al. "Food Intake and Immunologic Alteration in Mice
Fed Dehydroepiandrosterone." Experimental Gerontology.
1984, 19(5), pp. 297-304.

DMAE

DMAE, or dimethylaminoethanol, is normally present in small amounts in our brains. DMAE is known for its remarkable brain-enhancement effects. It is a naturally-occurring nutrient found in seafood such as anchovies and sardines. Perhaps this explains why fish has often been called brain food.

DMAE elevates mood, improves memory and learning, increases intelligence, extends life span of laboratory animals (Hochschild, 1978), and increases physical energy. It is used by many people for its mild, safe stimulant effect, and yet DMAE also makes it easier for most people to get to sleep. Many people report less fatigue in the day and sounder sleep at night as well as needing less sleep when taking DMAE.

The stimulant effect of DMAE is significantly different from the stimulation produced by coffee, amphetamines, or other stimulant drugs. DMAE does not have a drug-like quick up and quick come down. People who take DMAE have reported that after three to four weeks, they feel a mild stimulation continually, without side effects. Also, when DMAE is discontinued, no depression or let-down occurs.

Riker Laboratories developed a prescription drug called Deaner (also called Deanol). This substance is the p-acetamidobenzoate salt of DMAE and has very similar effects. Riker marketed their DMAE-like product for learning problems, under-achievement, shortened attention span, hyperactivity, reading and speech difficulties, impaired motor coordination, and behavior problems in children.

DMAE works by accelerating the brain's synthesis of the neurotransmitter acetylcholine, which in turn plays a key role in maximizing mental ability as well as in preventing loss of memory in aging adults.

Precautions: Overdosage can produce insomnia, dull head-aches, or tenseness in muscles (especially those of the jaws, neck, and legs). These side effects disappear if the dosage is lowered slightly. No serious adverse effects have ever been reported with DMAE. Patients with certain types of epilepsy should be closely monitored by a physician. DMAE should not be used by people who are manic depressive because it can deepen the depressive phase.

Dosage: DMAE is used initially at low dosages, with a gradual build up to 500mg or 1000mg per day. In some cases, lower dosages can result in a good response. DMAE can take as long as three weeks to take effect.

Sources: DMAE is considered a nutritional supplement and can be found at health food or drug stores. It comes in bulk powder form, capsules, or liquid. Liquid DMAE may spoil if left open or if stored at high temperatures. Keep it tightly sealed in the refrigerator. For sources of DMAE, see Appendix A (see page 165). Other names include: Acumen, Atrol, Atrol, Bimanol, Cervoxan, Deaner, Diforene, Dimethaen, dimethylaminoethanol, Elevan, Pabenol, Paxanol, Risatarun, Tonibral, and Varesal.

References:

Anderson, K., Anderson, L. **Orphan Drugs**. Los Angeles, CA: The Body Press, 1987, p. 69.

Ceder, G., et al. "Effects of 2-Dimethylaminoethanol (Deanol) on the Metabolism of Choline in Plasma." **Journal of Neurochemistry**. 1978, Vol. 30, pp. 1293-96.

Hochschild, R. "Effect of Dimethylaminoethyl p-Chlorophenoxy-acetate on the Life Span of Male Swiss Webster Albino Mice." **Experimental Gerontology**. 1973, Vol.8, pp. 177-83.

Honegger, C., Honegger, R. "Occurrence and Quantitative Determination of 2-Dimethylaminoethanol in Animal Tissue Extracts." **Nature**. 1959, Vol. 184, pp. 550-52.

Murphree, H.B., et al. "The Stimulant Effect of 2-Dimethylaminoethanol (Deanol) in Human Volunteer Subjects." **Clinical Pharmacology and Therapeutics**. 1960, Vol. 1, pp. 303-10.

Oettinger, L. "The Use of Deanol in the Treatment of Disorders of Behavior in Children." **The Journal of Pediatrics**. 1958, Vol. 3, pp. 671-5.

Osvaldo, R. "2-Dimethylaminoethanol (Deanol): A Brief Review of Its Clinical Efficacy and Postulated Mechanism of Action." **Current Therapeutic Research**. 1974, Vol. 16, No.11, pp. 1238-42.

Pearson, D., Shaw, S. **Life Extension: A Practical Scientific Approach**. New York: Warner Books, 1982.

Pelton, R., Pelton, T.C. **Mind Food & Smart Pills**. New York: Doubleday, 1989.

Pfeiffer, C.C. "Parasympathetic Neurohumors. Possible Precursors and Effect on Behavior." **International Review of Neurobiology**. 1959, pp. 195-244.

Pfeiffer, C.C., et al. "Stimulant Effect of 2-Dimethyl-l-aminoethanol: Possible Precursor of Brain Acetylcholine." **Science**. 1957, Vol. 126, pp. 610-1.

Zuckerman, B., Barrett, K."Effects of PCA and DMAE on the Nematode Caenorhabditis Briggsae." **Experimental Aging Research**. 1978, 4 (2) pp. 133-9.

Gerovital (GH-3)

Gerovital was developed in Romania in the 1940's by Dr. Ana Aslan at her government-sponsored geriatric clinic. Professor Aslan had been injecting procaine, a local anasthetic, into patients with painful arthritis, in order to relieve their joint pains. Many of her patients noted improved memory, less depression, more energy, restoration of normal hair color, improved skin tone, and a generalized feeling of well-being. These striking results encouraged her to carry out additional studies to test the effects of procaine on thousands of people. She found that by adding benzoic acid as a preservative, and potassium metabisulfite as an antioxidant, the procaine molecule was stabilized, and the effects were even more dramatic than with procaine alone. She called her "improved" form of procaine Gerovital or GH-3. She later added pyridoxine (vitamin B6), mesoinositol, and glutamic acid to procaine to form yet another version which she called Aslavital. Aslavital is claimed to have even greater effects than GH-3 on memory, atherosclerosis, and other degenerative conditions (Stroescu, 1988).

GH-3 is one of the most popular rejuvenation products in the world. GH-3 is also said by some researchers to be a powerful long-term antidepressant. Dr. Aslan's findings have been met with much skepticism, and studies done outside of Dr. Aslan's clinic have had mixed results.

Procaine in GH-3 is broken down in the body into the B vitamin PABA (para-aminobenzoic acid) and DEAE (diethyl-aminoethanol). The DEAE molecule is very similar to DMAE (see the section on DMAE) and has some similar effects.

GH-3 has been shown to inhibit an enzyme called mono-amine oxidase (MAO), an enzyme in the brain. MAO breaks down monoamine neurotransmitters like dopamine, serotonin, and norepinephrine. As people get older, MAO activity increases, breaking down these neurotransmitters too rapidly. Dopamine, serotonin, and norepinephrine trigger feelings of pleasure, serenity, and calmness. People using GH-3 report increased energy levels, alertness, and improvement in mood. These effects may be due to the MAO-inhibiting action of GH-3.

One study showed that procaine improved oxygen utilization in the brains of old rats to levels that were equal to those in young rats, suggesting that this may be another way that GH-3 accomplishes its effects.

GH-3 is approved by the Romanian equivalent of the U.S. FDA for treatment of "old age phenomenon", to include neuritis, neuralgia, cerebral and peripheral atherosclerosis, Parkinson's disease, and arthritis, among others. Recent studies have reported GH-3's effectiveness in a number of conditions, including mental retardation in children (Aslan, 1980a; Aslan, 1980b), Parkinson's disease (Aslan, 1982), and Alzheimer's disease (Vlachou-Economou, 1988). Several studies have compared the efficacy of GH-3 with piracetam, resulting in similar improvements in central nervous system functioning (Stroescu, 1985; Stroescu, 1986). A third study resulted in even greater improvements in cognitive functioning when piracetam was combined with Aslavital (Stroescu, 1986).

Other studies have failed to replicate these findings about GH-3. Many of the studies which claim to discredit GH-3 used straight procaine rather than the GH-3 preparation from Romania. The researchers believed, for good reasons, that procaine is identical to GH-3. The developers of GH-3 however, claim that the trace amounts of other ingredients are significant.

Precautions: There are no reports of serious negative effects of GH-3, except rare allergic reactions.

Dosage: One GH-3 tablet is taken daily for 25 days. Then no tablets are taken for five days before another round is begun. In its injectable form, GH-3 is used every third day for a month, then rest for one month before beginning another round. This complicated schedule was devised by Dr. Aslan to allow the restorations of enzymes necessary to break down procaine, and to "desensitize" the body to the effects of procaine. This schedule is too difficult for many patients to follow. One to two injections per week on a continuing basis seem to provide equivalent benefit.

Sources: In the U.S. GH-3 can only be purchased in Nevada. It is available over the counter in Romania, most European countries, and Mexico or by mail order from the sources listed in Appendix A (see page 165). Other names include: Gerontex H3, Gerovital, Gerovital H3, KH3, and Sex-Ex.

References:

"Gerovital-H3: The Youth Drug." **Anti-Aging News**. January 1981, p. 2.

Aslan, A., et al. "Long-term Treatment with Procaine (Gerovital-H3) in Albino Rats." **Journal of Gerontology**. 1965, Vol. 20, p. 1.

Aslan, A. "The Therapeutics of Old Age: The Action of Procaine." Blumethal, H. T., ed., **Medical and Clinical Aspects of Aging**. New York: Columbia University Press, 1962.

Aslan, A., Balaceanu, C., Manoiu, A., Erdos, M., Konig, V., et al. "The Effects of Gerovital H3 Treatment in Parkinsonian Syndromes." **Romanian Journal of Gerontology and Geriatrics**. 1982, 3: 3, pp. 201-213.

Aslan, A., Vrabiescu, A., Dobre, M. "Aslavital for Children in Mentally Deficient Subjects." **Romanian Journal of Gerontology and Geriatrics**. 1980, 1: 2, pp. 189-194.

Aslan, A., Vrabiescu, A., Dobre, M., Polovrageany, E. "The Aslavital Treatment in the Recovery of Mentally-Deficient Children." **Romanian Journal of Gerontology and Geriatrics**. 1980, 1: 1, pp. 93-98.

Bailey, H. **GH-3**. New York: Bantam Books. 1977, pp. 284-85.

Ostfeld, A., Smith, C.M., Stotsky, B.A. "The Systemic Use of Procaine in the Treatment of the Elderly: A Review." **Journal of the American Geriatrics Society**. January 1977, Vol. 25, pp. 1-19.

Pearson, D., Shaw, S. **Life Extension: A Practical Scientific Approach**. New York: Warner Books, 1982.

Pelton, R., Pelton, T.C. **Mind Food & Smart Pills**. New York: Doubleday, 1989.

Samorajski, T., Rolstein, C. "Effects of Chronic Dosage with Chlorpromazine and Gerovital-H3 in the Aging Brain." **Aging Brain & Senile Dementia**. New York: Plenum Press, 1976.

Smigel, J.O., et al. "H3 (Procaine Hydrochloride) Therapy in Aging Institutionalized Patients: An Interim Report." **Journal of American Gerontological Society**. 1960, Vol. 8, p. 785.

Stroescu, V. "The Experimental and Clinical Pharmacology of Procaine, Gerovital H3 and Aslavital." **Romanian Journal of Gerontology and Geriatrics**. 1988, 9: 4, pp. 427-437.

Stroescu, V., Constantinescu, I., Brezina, A., Hamzeh, B., Vrabiescu, A. "Experimental Studies on the Nootropic Effects Exerted

Upon the Central Nervous System by Gerovital H3 Versus Procaine and Pyracetam." **Romanian Journal of Gerontology and Geriatrics**. 1985, 6: 2, pp. 105-111.

Stroescu, V., Constantinescu, I., Brezina, A., Niculcea-Lungulescu, A., Vrabiescu, A. "Experimental Trial on the Combined Action of Procaine and Pyracetam Upon the Central Nervous System." **Romanian Journal of Gerontology and Geriatrics**. 1989, 10: 2, pp. 105-115.

Stroescu, V., Constantinescu, I., Brezina, A., Sotirescu, D. "Experimental Studies into the Nootropic Effects Exerted Upon the Central Nervous System by Aslavital Versus Procaine and Pyracetam." **Romanian Journal of Gerontology and Geriatrics**. 1986, 7: 2, pp. 115-121.

Thomas, R. "Procaine. Will It Keep You Younger Longer?" **The Medical Journal of Australia**. June 11, 1983, pp. 543-5.

Verzar, F. "Note on the Influence of Procaine, PABA, and DEAE on the Aging of Rats." **Gerontologia**. 1959, Vol. 3, p. 351.

Vlachou-Economou, S. "Clinical and Therapeutical Researches with Aslavital Long-Term Treatment in Alzheimer's Disease." **Romanian Journal of Gerontology and Geriatrics**. 1988, 9: Supplement 1, p. 47.

Walford, R.L. **Maximum Life Span**. New York: W.W. Norton, 1983.

Zwerling, I. "Effects of a Procaine Preparation (Gerovital-H3) in Hospitalized Geriatric Patients: A Double Blind Study." **Journal of American Gerontological Society**. Vol. 23, p. 8.

Ginkgo Biloba: A Nootropic Herb?

Ginkgo biloba is the oldest species of tree known, dating back 300 million years. Extracts from the leaves of the ginkgo biloba tree have been used in Chinese medicine for thousands of years. Today, European physicians write over 1.2 million prescriptions per month for it. Ginkgo biloba is used to improve cerebral circulation, mental alertness, and overall brain functioning.

More than 34 human studies on ginkgo have been published since 1975, showing that ginkgo leaf works by increasing blood flow throughout the body and brain. Ginkgo increases the production of adenosine triphosphate (ATP, the universal energy molecule). It also improves the brain's ability to metabolize glucose, prevents platelet aggregation inside arterial walls by keeping them flexible, improves the transmission of nerve signals, and acts as a powerful antioxidant.

Ginkgo biloba leaf is effective for people with symptoms of reduced blood flow to the brain and extremities. It has been shown to be helpful with many of the complaints of the elderly such as: short-term memory loss, slow thinking and reasoning, depression, dizziness, ringing in the ears, headaches, and senile macular degeneration (a major cause of blindness).

One study even shows significant improvement in people

who have both Parkinson's *and* Alzheimer's disease. In this study 25 people with Parkinson's and signs of Alzheimer's disease were given ginkgo extract daily for one year. They were tested with standard tests, clinical evaluations, and a new computerized EEG. The scores improved significantly (Funfgeld, 1989).

One study does not prove that Ginkgo biloba is efficacious in the treatment of these diseases. However, ginkgo is safe, inexpensive and easily obtained, and people with Parkinson's and/or Alzheimer's disease might consider experimenting with it.

One researcher believes Ginkgo Biloba belongs in the class of compounds known as "nootropics", even though it is from an herbal source.

Precautions: No negative effects have been reported in the literature even at very large quantities.

Dosage: Most research has been done with a ginkgo biloba extract which contained a 24% concentration of flavonoid extract. At this strength, the usual dosage is 120-160mg per day taken in three divided doses. However, many ginkgo products on the market are lower in potency. These products are taken in dosages as high as 1000mg per day in three divided doses. Three to six months use is probably needed to evaluate the results.

Sources: Ginkgo biloba leaf and extracts are available in vitamin and health food stores. Source Naturals is one company that has a good ginkgo biloba leaf extract. They have a product called "Ginkgo-24" with 40mg of 24.3%

ginkgo flavone glycosides per tablet. See Appendix A (page 165) for other sources.

References:

Allard, M. "Treatment of Old Age Disorders with Ginkgo Biloba Extract." **La Presse Medicale**. 1986, Vol. 15, No. 31, p. 1540.

Auguet, M., Delaflotte, S., Hellegouarch, A., Clostre, F. "Bases Pharmacologiques de l'Impact Vasculaire de l'Extrait de Ginkgo Biloba," **La Presse Medicale**. 1986, Vol. 15, No. 31, p. 1524.

Funfgeld, E.W. "A Natural and Broad Spectrum Nootropic Substance for Treatment of SDAT—the Ginkgo Biloba Extract." **Progress in Clinical and Biological Research**. 1989, 317, pp. 1247-60.

Gebner, B., Voelp, A., Klasser, M. "Study of the Long-term Action of a Ginkgo Biloba Extract on Vigilance and Mental Performance as Determined by Means of Quantitative Pharmaco-EEG and Psychometric Measurements." **Arzneimittelforschung**. 1985, Vol. 35, No. 9, pp. 1459-65.

Hindmarch, I. "Activity of Ginkgo Biloba Extract on Short-term Memory." **La Presse Medicale**. 1986, Vol. 15, No. 31, p. 1562, 1592.

Pelton, R., Pelton, T.C. **Mind Food & Smart Pills**. New York: Doubleday, 1989.

Schaffler, K., Reeh, P. "Long-term Drug Administration Effects of Ginkgo Biloba on the Performance of Healthy Subjects Exposed to Hypoxia." From Agnoli, J., **Effects of Ginkgo Biloba Extracts on Organic Cerebral Impairment**. Eurotext Ltd., 1985, pp. 77-84.

Taillandier, J., Ammar, A., Rabourdin, J.P., Ribeyre, J.P., Pichon, J., Niddam, S., Pierart, H. "Traitement des Troubles du Viellissement Cerebral par l'Extract de Ginkgo Biloba." **La Presse Medicale**. 1986, Vol. 15, No. 31. p. 1583.

Warburton, D.M. "Clinical Psychopharmacology of Ginkgo Biloba Extract." **La Presse Medicale**. 1986, Vol. 15, No. 31, p. 1595.

Ginseng

Unlike drugs which are designed to act against a specific disease or symptom, ginseng has a wide range of uses. Ginseng appears to function by acting as an adaptogen, a nontoxic substance that increases resistance to stress. Adaptogens have a remarkable ability to normalize conditions in the body, restoring homeostasis, and protecting against stress and fatigue.

Ginseng improves brain function, concentration, memory and learning. In addition, it can reduce or normalize heart beat, blood sugar, and cholesterol, stimulate metabolic functions, and increase endocrine activity. Ginseng can stimulate the circulatory system and digestion, quench free radicals, increase resistance to drugs, alcohol, chemotherapy, and other toxins. It is known to improve athletic performance, shorten recovery time after exercise or stressful situations, benefit insomnia and sleep disturbances, stimulate the immune system, and improve sexual function. It is ginseng's ability to normalize conditions in the body that give it this rather long list of benefits.

The medicinal properties of ginseng appear to be due to a group of chemicals called saponins, also known as glycosides or ginsenosides. These chemicals influence the metabolism of neurotransmitters like serotonin and acetylcholine, which are important for optimum mental functioning. Ginseng seems to reduce the activation of the adrenal cortex, and therefore inhibits the alarm stage of stress. Saponins also increase the activity of the lymphocytes, enhancing immune function. Many of the effects of ginseng are due to its ability to regulate the energy in your body and brain.

Precautions: Individuals with high blood pressure should be cautious about using large quantities of ginseng. In Chinese medicine, there are "types" for whom ginseng is contraindicated. Also, Chinese medicine uses ginseng as a tonic, not necessarily on a daily basis.

Dosage: 500mg to 3000mg per day in divided doses.

Sources: Most health food stores carry several varieties of ginseng. There is tremendous variation in the amount of active ingredients found in different types of ginseng and ginseng products. For sources of ginseng see Appendix A on page 165.

References:

Baburin, E.F. "On the Effect of Eleutherococcus Senticosus on the Results of Work and Hearing Acuity of Radio-Telegraphers." Brekham, I.I., ed., **Eleutherococcus and Other Adaptogens Among the Far Eastern Plants**. Vladivostok, U.S.S.R.: Far Eastern Publishing House. 1966, pp. 179-84.

Brekham, I.I. **Eleutherococcus**. Leningrad: Nauka Publishing House. 1968.

Fulder, S. "The Drug That Builds Russians." **New Scientist**, 1980.

Ginseng, Ten of the Most Commonly Asked Questions About the Root of Life. International Health Publications, 1977 (pamphlet).

"Ginseng: The Anti-Stress Therapy." **Anti-Aging News.** October 1983, p. 111.

Iljutjecok, R.J., Tjaplygina, S.R. "The Effect of a Preparation of Eleutherococcus Senticosus on Memory in Mice." The Department of Physiology, Academy of Sciences of the Soviet Union, Novosibirsk. 1978.

Pelton, R., Pelton, T.C. **Mind Food & Smart Pills.** New York: Doubleday, 1989.

Petkov, V., Staneua, S. "The Effect of an Extract of Ginseng on the Adrenal Cortex." **Proceedings of the 2nd International Pharmacology Meeting.** Prague, 1963. New York: Pergamon Press. Vol. 7, pp. 39-45.

Petkov, V. "Effects of Standardized Ginseng Extract on Learning, Memory and Physical Capabilities." **American Journal of Chinese Medicine.** 1987, Vol. 15, No. 1, pp. 19-29.

Petkov, V. **Pharmazeutische Zeitung.** 1968, Vol. 31.

Quiroga, H.A., Imbriano, A.E. "The Effect of Panax Ginseng Extract on Cerebrovascular Deficits." **Orientacion Medica.** 1979, Vol. 28: 1208, pp. 86-7.

Seigel, R.D. "Ginseng Abuse Syndrome." **Journal of the American Medical Association.** 1979.

Voskersarsky, T., et al. "Effect of Eleutherococcus and Ginseng on the Development of Free-Radical Pathology." **Proceeding of the Second International Symposium of Eleutherococcus.** Moscow, 1985, pp. 141-45.

Hydergine

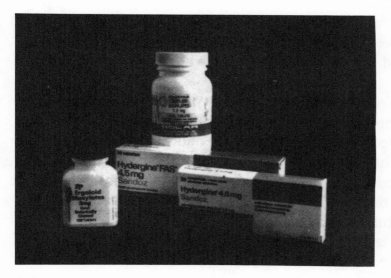

Hydergine is reported to increase mental abilities, prevent damage to brain cells from insufficient oxygen (hypoxia), and may even be able to reverse existing damage to brain cells.

Hydergine is an extract of ergot, a fungus that grows on rye. Midwives in Europe traditionally used ergot with birthing mothers to lower their blood pressure. Researchers at the pharmaceutical giant Sandoz analyzed ergot in the late 1940s, looking for blood-pressure medications. Of the thousands of compounds that researchers found in ergot, three were combined and tested for their anti-hypertensive properties. When studies with elderly people uncovered cognition-enhancing effects, Sandoz began spending a great deal of research money on Hydergine. It is now one of the most popular treatments for all forms of senility in the U.S., and is used to treat a plethora of problems elsewhere in the world.

Hydergine probably has several modes of action for its cognitive-enhancement properties. Its wide variety of reported effects include the following:

1) Increases blood supply and oxygen to the brain.
2) Enhances brain cell metabolism.
3) Protects the brain from free-radical damage during decreased or increased oxygen supply.
4) Speeds the elimination of age pigment (lipofuscin) in the brain.
5) Inhibits free-radical activity.
6) Increases intelligence, memory, learning, and recall.
7) Normalizes systolic blood pressure.
8) Lowers abnormally high cholesterol levels in some cases.
9) Reduces symptoms of tiredness.
10) Reduces symptoms of dizziness and tinnitus (ringing in the ears).

In their landmark book, *Life Extension: A Practical Scientific Approach*, Durk Pearson and Sandy Shaw called Hydergine "the most tested pharmaceutical ever invented." Hydergine has been proven to be beneficial and nontoxic in research project after research project.

One way that Hydergine may enhance memory and learning is by mimicking the effect of a substance called nerve growth factor (NGF). NGF stimulates protein synthesis, resulting in the growth of dendrites (tiny extensions which branch out from brain cells making connections with other brain cells). Dendrites are the communication connections between nerve and brain cells and are crucial to memory and learning.

Hydergine was the first drug to show efficacy against Alzheimer's disease (Branconnier, 1983). The efficacy of Hydergine in dementias is as well-proven as almost any drug used for treating psychiatric disorders (Hollister, 1988). At the time of a 1979 review, more than 20 double-blind placebo-controlled trials had been conducted to test Hydergine with senile dementias. All noted statistically significant improvements in behavioral and psychological parameters. Numerous favorable studies have been published since then. One recent study, however, reported no improvement in 39 Alzheimer's patients who were treated with 1mg Hydergine three times per day for six months (Thompson, 1990). These negative results may be due to the disease having progressed beyond help, or perhaps because an inadequate dosage of Hydergine was used. In an earlier study of patients with multi-infarct dementias or mental disturbances following strokes, Yoshikawa and his colleagues (1983) demonstrated that a six-mg-per-day dose was far superior to the standard three-mg-per-day dose. The literature suggests that Hydergine treatment be started early in Alzheimer's patients.

Precautions: If too large a dose is used when first taking Hydergine, it may cause slight nausea, gastric disturbance, or headache. Overall, Hydergine does not produce any serious side effects. It is nontoxic even at very large doses and it is contraindicated only for individuals who have chronic or acute psychosis, or who are allergic to it. Overdosage of Hydergine may, paradoxically, cause an amnesic effect.

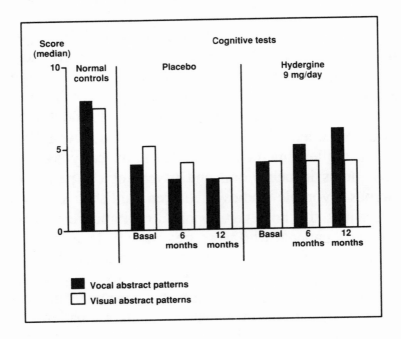

*Change in abstract thought patterns in Alzheimer's patients on placebo or high doses of Hydergine. Placebo-treated patients show progressive deterioration, while Hydergine patients show improvement on tests of vocal abstract patterns and remain stable on tests of visual abstract patterns. (Redrawn from **Age-Related Mental Decline and Dementias, The Place of Hydergine,** Sandoz product literature booklet.)*

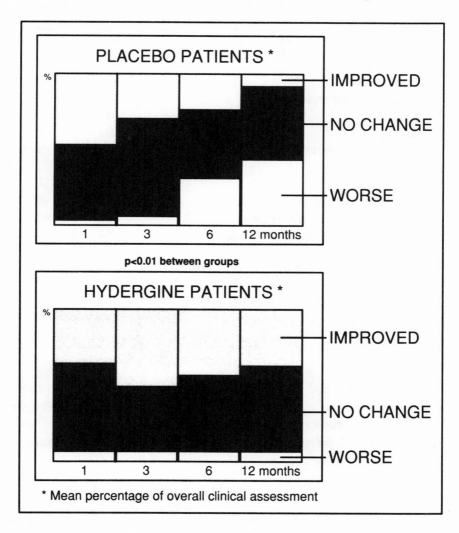

*Assessment by families of patients with cerebral insufficiency. (Redrawn from **The Three Early Symptoms Pointing to Cerebral Insufficiency**, Sandoz product literature.)*

Symptoms	Hydergine%	Placebo%
Hostility	**86**	**41**
Dizziness	**77**	**58**
Bothersomeness	**69**	**58**
Irritability	**67**	**48**
Confusion	**64**	**28**
Uncooperativeness	**64**	**40**
Mood-depression	**61**	**32**
Unsociability	**60**	**30**
Impaired recent memory	**60**	**40**
Impaired mental alertness	**56**	**40**
Indifference to surroundings	**54**	**44**
Anorexia	**54**	**23**
Anxiety	**54**	**54**
Impaired self-care	**50**	**30**
Impaired motivation and initiative	**48**	**36**
Emotional lability	**44**	**34**
Fatigue	**40**	**25**

Subjects (average age of 77) with moderately impaired behavioral and cognitive functioning were given 3mg per day of Hydergine or placebo for 12 weeks. The graph represents percentages of patients who improved. (Redrawn from **Hydergine Tablets: General Summary of Information,** *Medical Services Department, Sandoz Pharmaceuticals, 1978.)*

Dosage: The U.S. recommended dosage is 3 mg per day. However, the European recommended dosage is 9 mg per day taken in three divided doses. It may take several months before you notice the effects of Hydergine.

The effects of Hydergine may be synergistic with piracetam. If you are taking both you may need to scale down the dosage of both smart drugs in order to get the optimal cognitive enhancing effect. Since these and many of the compounds we discuss have inverted "U" dose response curves you might even get a reverse effect if you take high doses of piracetam and Hydergine together. Please see The Use of Cerebroactive Substances for more on synergistic effects.

Sources: Hydergine is available in the U.S. with a doctor's prescription. Keep in mind, however, that your doctor may not be familiar with the uses we have discussed. Hydergine can also be purchased over the counter in Mexico or by mail order from the sources listed in Appendix A (see page 165). Other names for Hydergine include: Circanol, Coristin, D-Ergotox forte L.U.T., Dacoren, Deapril-ST, Decme, Decril, Defluina, DHE, DHET, dihydroergotoxine, Dulcion, Enirant, Ergodesit, Ergohydrin, ergoloid mesylates, Ergoplus, Insibrin, Nehydrin, Novofluen, Orphol, Perenan, Progeril, Redergin, Simactil, Sponsin, Trigot, and Unergol.

References:

Branconnier, R. "The Efficacy of the Cerebral Metabolic Enhancers in the Treatment of Senile Dementia." **Psychopharmacology Bulletin**. 1983, 19(2), pp. 212-20.

Copeland, R.L., Jr., Bhattacharyya, A.K., Aulakh, C.S., Pradhan, S.N. "Behavioral and Neurochemical Effects of Hydergine in Rats." **Archives of International Pharmacodynamics**. 1981, Vol. 252, pp. 113-23.

Emmenegger, H., Meier-Ruge, W. "The Actions of Hydergine on the Brain." **Pharmacology**. 1968, Vol. 1, pp. 65-78.

Exton-Smith, A.N., et al. "Clinical Experience with Ergot Alkaloids." **Aging**. New York: Raven Press, 1983, Vol. 23, p. 323.

Fanchamps, A. "Dihydroergotoxine in Senile Cerebral Insufficiency." **Aging**. New York: Raven Press, 1983, Vol. 23, pp. 311-22.

Hindmarch, I., Parrott, A.C., Lanza, M. "The Effects of an Ergot Alkaloid Derivative (Hydergine) on Aspects of Psychomotor

Performance, Arousal, and Cognitive Processing Ability." **The Journal of Clinical Pharmacology.** November-December 1979, pp. 726-31.

Hollister, L.E. "Ergoloid Mesylates and the Treatment of Senile Dementias." **Perspectives in Psychopharmacology: A Collection of Papers in Honor of Earl Usdin.** 1988, New York, Alan R. Liss, pp. 613-20.

Hughes, J.R., Williams, J.G., Currier, R.D. "An Ergot Alkaloid Preparation (Hydergine) in the Treatment of Dementia: A Critical Review of the Clinical Literature." **Journal of the American Geriatrics Society.** 1976, Vol. 24, pp. 490-97.

Pearson, D., Shaw, S. **Life Extension: A Practical Scientific Approach.** New York: Warner Books, 1982.

Pelton, R., Pelton, T.C. **Mind Food & Smart Pills.** New York: Doubleday, 1989.

Rao, D.B., Norris, J.R. "A Double-Blind Investigation of Hydergine in the Treatment of Cerebrovascular Insufficiency in the Elderly." **Johns Hopkins Medical Journal.** 1971, Vol. 130, pp. 317-23.

Spiegel, R., Huber, F., Koberle, S. "A Controlled Long-Term Study with Ergoloid Mesylates (Hydergine) in Healthy, Elderly Volunteers: Results After Three Years." **Journal of the Geriatrics Society.** 1983, Vol. 31, No. 9, pp. 549-55.

Thompson, T.L. II, Filley, C.M., Mitchell, W.D., et al. "Lack of Efficacy of Hydergine in Patients with Alzheimer's Disease." **New England Journal of Medicine.** 1990, 323: pp. 445-8.

Weil, C., ed. "Pharmacology and Clinical Pharmacology of Hydergine." **Handbook of Experimental Pharmacology.** New York: Springer-Verlag, 1978.

Yesavage, J.A., Hollister, L.E., Burian, E. "Dihydroergotoxine: 6-Mg versus 3-Mg Dosage in the Treatment of Senile Dementia. Preliminary Report." **Journal of the American Geriatrics Society.** 1979, Vol. 27, No. 2, pp. 80-82.

Yoshikawa, M., Hirai, S., Aizawa, T., Kuroiwa, Y., Goto, F., Sofue, I., Toyokura, Y., Yamamura, H., Iwasaki, Y. "A Dose-Response Study with Dihydroergotoxine Mesylate in Cerebrovascular Disturbances." **Journal of the American Geriatrics Society.** 1983, Vol. 31, No. 1, pp. 1-7.

Idebenone

Idebenone is closely related to CoEnzyme Q_{10} (CoQ$_{10}$), a substance that has been assiduously studied in Japan. CoQ$_{10}$ is an important biological molecule, and is found in very high concentrations in the human heart. It has a key role in the creation of ATP, the universal energy molecule. CoQ$_{10}$ has many remarkable properties, including extending life span in animals, and curing some gum diseases in humans

Coenzyme Q$_{10}$

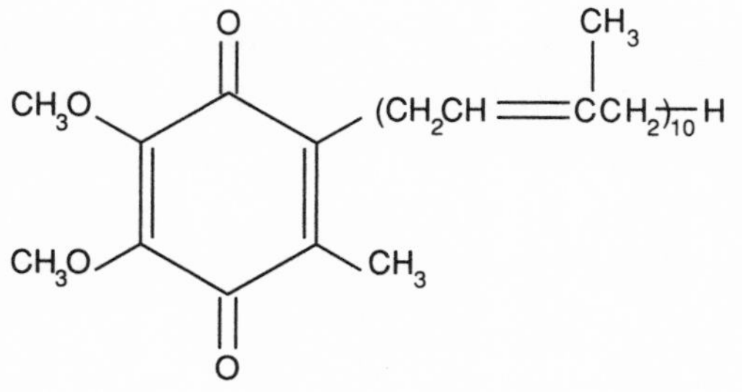

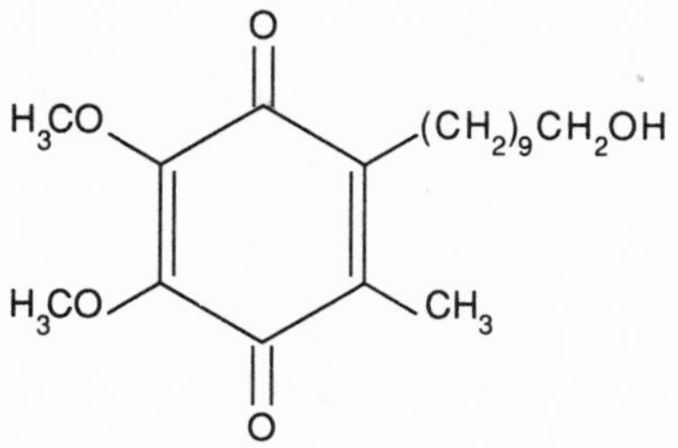

CH$_3$O $\quad$ (CH$_2$CH$=$CCH$_2$)$_{10}$H

CH$_3$O $\quad$ CH$_3$

H$_3$CO $\quad$ (CH$_2$)$_9$CH$_2$OH

H$_3$CO $\quad$ CH$_3$

Idebenone

more effectively than any other substance. However, CoQ_{10} has troubled some researchers because of its ability to metabolize into a toxic molecule with a highly reactive free radical. Idebenone seems to have all the benefits of CoQ_{10}, yet it does not create such a reactive metabolite (Pearson and Shaw, 1989).

Idebenone is an antioxidant. It can reduce the damage caused by strokes induced in experimental animals. It also improves cerebral energy metabolism.

Idebenone protects experimental animals from the debilitating effects on memory and cognition caused by hypoxia (deficient blood oxygenation), anti-cholinergic substances, and low levels of the neurotransmitter serotonin.

Low serotonin levels were induced in rats to test the effects of idebenone. The rats were fed diets with no tryptophan, a precursor of serotonin. When given idebenone, the rats performed as well on a discrimination test as rats with normal serotonin levels (Nomura, 1985). Another study, on seven patients with mental and intellectual impairment, showed that idebenone can improve neurotransmitter levels in patients with cerebrovascular dementia, especially promoting serotonin replacement (Kawakami, 1989). Low serotonin levels in humans are associated with impulsiveness, bad temper and violent behavior. Studies of violent people in prisons have found low levels of serotonin metabolites, indicating low serotonin levels. If you fly off the handle too easily, idebenone could have profound stabilizing effects on your state of mind. We would appreciate hearing from anyone who experiments with idebenone for this purpose.

Precautions: The one safety/tolerance study we could find said that idebenone, "was well-tolerated with regard to the subjective and objective assessments made during the study. There were no changes in clinical laboratory values which could be directly attributed to the administration of idebenone" (Barkworth, 1985).

Dosage: 100mg per day.

Sources: Idebenone is available in Japan with a doctor's prescription, but is very expensive. Other names include: Avan and CV-2619.

References:

Barkworth, M.F., Dyde, C.J., Johnson, K.I., Schnelle, K. "An Early Phase I Study to Determine the Tolerance, Safety and Pharmacokinetics of Idebenone Following Multiple Oral Doses." **Arzneimittelforschung**. 1985, 35 (11) pp. 1704-7.

Kawakami, M., Itoh, T. "Effects of Idebenone on Monoamine Metabolites in Cerebrospinal Fluid of Patients with Cerebrovascular Dementia." **Archives of Gerontology and Geriatrics**. 1989, 8 (3) pp. 343-53.

Kiyota, Y., Miyamoto, M., Nagaoka, A. "Ameliorating Effects of Idebenone and Indeloxazine Hydrochloride on Impairment of Radial Maze Learning in Cerebral Embolized Rats." **Nippon Yakurigaku Zasshi**. 1989, 93 (3) pp. 197-202.

Nomura, M. "Effect of Idebenone (CV-2619) on Brightness Discrimination Learning in Rats with Central Serotonergic Dysfunction." **Yakubutsu Seishin Kodo**. 1985, 5 (3) pp. 243-9.

Pearson, D., Shaw, S. **Durk Pearson & Sandy Shaw's Life Extension Newsletter**. September-October 1989, Vol 2, Number 7, p. 62.

Yamazaki, N., Nomura, M., Nagaoka, A., Nagawa, Y. "Idebenone Improves Learning and Memory Impairment Induced by Cholinergic or Serotonergic Dysfunction in Rats." **Archives of Gerontology and Geriatrics**. 1989, 8 (3) pp. 225-39.

Phenytoin (Dilantin)

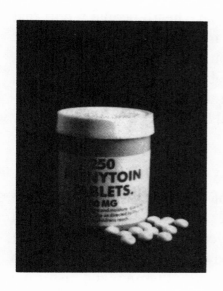

Dilantin is known to most doctors and many other people as a treatment for epilepsy. However, it has a wide range of pharmacologic effects other than its anticonvulsant activity. There have been more than 8,000 papers published on Dilantin and there have been clinical reports of its usefulness in over 100 diseases and symptoms (Finkel, 1984).

In the United States the only officially-approved uses for Dilantin are for controlling various types of seizures.

Dilantin has an extraordinary ability to stabilize electrical activity at the cell membrane. Since most cellular activity is modulated by the electrical and electro-chemical processes that occur on the cell membranes, Dilantin has a host of effects and uses.

Dilantin is reported to increase intelligence, concentration, and learning. In double-blind, placebo-controlled studies, 100mg of Dilantin given twice daily caused increases in

129

scores on the Wechsler IQ test and improved long term memory and verbal performance in both normal, healthy young and normal, healthy elderly volunteers. Particular improvement was noted by researchers in the subject's performance on parts of the tests requiring concentration skills (Smith, 1972, 1975). We have heard people report that Dilantin is a fast and effective treatment for jet lag, lack of sleep, or any situation where you need more stamina. Several thousand research studies have been conducted on Dilantin, establishing its effectiveness in the treatment of drug addiction, alcoholism, psychosis, and hypoglycemia, to name only a few.

Dilantin is of special interest to people who cannot concentrate or think clearly because of obsessive thoughts, or who experience a lot of fear or anger. Research done with prison inmates and institutionalized juvenile delinquents showed that Dilantin decreases violent behavior. Also, in subjects who were overly passive, it increased outgoing and assertive behavior. Dilantin seems to have a normalizing effect (Dreyfus, 1981).

The Dilantin story is told in a book by Jack Dreyfus, the wealthy philanthropist who started the Dreyfus Fund. In *A Remarkable Medicine Has Been Overlooked*, Dreyfus recounts how he stumbled onto Dilantin as a treatment for his obsessive depression. He tells of the subsequent founding of the Dreyfus Medical Foundation, to spread the word about the many uses for Dilantin.

Dreyfus' descriptions of his own depression and obsessive fear and anxiety are moving, and occasionally hilarious. He describes being unable to work, and being obsessed about events such as animals he has seen killed by automobiles on the road. Dreyfus writes of worrying about a girl that he met at a party, the daughter of a famous actress. He feared that the 17-year-old would fail in her attempt to follow in her mother's footsteps, and worried about her obsessively for days, even though he had only met her briefly. The girl was Liza Minelli.

Jack Dreyfus' life was changed completely by Dilantin, and he became curious about other uses for it. His medical foundation spent $6 million researching and attempting to communicate the many uses of Dilantin.

Dilantin also has profound anti-aging effects, acting to restore neuroendocrine homeostasis that is inevitably lost with aging (Dilman and Dean, 1992). In low doses, it increases levels of protective high density lipoprotein (HDL)—the "good" form of cholesterol (Kaste, 1978).

Precautions: Like many of the smart drugs in this book, Dilantin can have paradoxical effects if too much is taken. Epileptics who must take very large doses of Dilantin show a slowing of reaction time and a reduction in intelligence. Dilantin may also cause a marked reduction in the body's B-12 stores (Newbold, 1972), and increase the body's requirement for thyroid hormone (Dilman and Dean, 1992). There are also some deleterious long term effects of Dilantin such as gum overgrowth. This effect is not likely to occur with someone who is taking the much lower cognitive-enhancing doses. The gum-overgrowing tendency can also be greatly relieved by meticulous oral hygiene, to include diligently flossing the teeth and rinsing the mouth with hydrogen peroxide. Dilantin should not be used by pregnant women, or people with cardiac or renal problems.

Dosage: For the treatment of epilepsy, the standard adult dosage is 200mg - 400mg per day in 2 to 4 divided doses. For cognition-enhancing purposes much smaller doses like 25 or 50mg per day are probably sufficient. Dilantin is available in 100mg capsules, 50mg children's chewable tablets, and a liquid containing 125mg of dilantin per teaspoon.

Sources: Dilantin is available in the U.S. with a doctor's prescription or from the overseas sources listed in Appendix A (see page 165). Other names for Dilantin include: Alepsin, Aleviatan, Antisacer, Citrullamon, Danten, Denyl Sodium, Derizene, Di-Len, Di-Lan, Di-Hydan, Difhydan, Dihycon, Dilabid, Diphenine Sodium, Diphentoin, Diphenylan Sodium, diphenylhydantoin, DPH, Ekko, Epamin, Epanutin, Epanutin, Eplin, Eptoin, Hidantal, Hydantol, Idantoin, Lehydan, Lepitoin Sodium, Minetoin, Phenhydan, Phenhydan, phenytoin, Solantoin, Solantyl, Tacosal, Thilophenyt, and Zentropil.

References:

Dilman, V.M., Dean, W. **The Neuroendocrine Theory of Aging and Degenerative Disease**. Pensacola, Florida: The Center for Bio-Gerontology, 1992.
Dreyfus, J. **A Remarkable Medicine Has Been Overlooked**. New York: Simon and Schuster, 1981.
Finkel, M.J. "Phenytoin Revisited." **Journal of Clinical Therapeutics**. 1984, 6 (5), pp. 577-91.
Gibbs, M.E., Ng, K.T. "Diphenylhydantoin Extension of Short-Term and Intermediate Stages of Memory." **Behavior and Brain Research**. 1984, 11 (2) pp. 103-8.
Gibbs, M.E., Ng. K.T. "Diphenylhydantoin Facilitation of Labile, Protein Independent Memory." **Brain Research Bulletin**. 1976, 1 (2) pp. 203-8.
Kaste, M. "Elevation of High-Density Lipoprotein in Epileptic Patients

Treated with Phenytoin." **Acta Medica Scandinavica.** 1978, 204: pp. 517-520.

Newbold, H. "The Use of Vitamin B-12 in Psychiatric Practice." **Orthomolecular Psychiatry,** Vol 1, No 1, 1972.

Pelton, R., Pelton, T.C. **Mind Food & Smart Pills.** New York Doubleday, 1989.

Smith, W., Lowry, J. "The Effects of Diphenylhydantoin on Cognitive Functions in Man." **Drugs, Development and Cerebral Function.** Springfield, IL: Charles C. Thomas, 1972, pp. 344-351.

Smith, W., Lowry, J. "Effects of Diphenylhydantoin on Mental Abilities in the Elderly." **Journal of the American Geriatric Society.** 1975, Vol. 23, 5, pp. 207-11.

Propranolol Hydrochloride (Inderal)

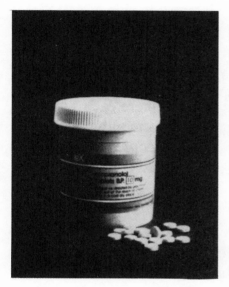

Propranolol hydrochloride was for many years the most prescribed drug in the U.S. It is usually prescribed for the control of high blood pressure. However, it has one effect that in some situations can be thought of as intelligence-increasing.

Propranolol blocks the receptor site for adrenaline in the muscles. Adrenaline is often referred to as the "flight or fight" neurotransmitter. This means that fear (such as stage fright) can cause the body to release enormous amounts of adrenaline into the blood stream. This was a very effective bio-chemical strategy when most fear-producing situations called for fighting or fleeing. Unfortunately, fighting and fleeing are of little help when one is giving a presentation to the board of directors, taking an important exam, going out on a blind date, or attending a social gathering with important and intimidating strangers.

Fear causes the body to spiral into an ever-increasing loop: more adrenaline causes more fear, which causes more adrenaline, etc. Propranolol can help. Blocking adrenaline interrupts the fear spiral. So propranolol is an intelligence-increasing drug when used in situations where fear prevents one from thinking normally.

Propranolol has one more very interesting side effect: if it is used on three or four different occasions in a situation that normally causes fear, you may no longer need to use it in that situation. For example, you may have a new job that requires you to give weekly speeches. If the speeches are in the same room and the same people are there each time, you will probably not need propranolol after a month or so. If the fear situation involves new places and people, the effects of propranolol may not generalize this quickly, if at all.

Precautions: Propranolol lowers blood pressure. People with hypotension (abnormally low blood pressure) should not use propranolol. Always take propranolol with food or it may cause nausea, especially if taken with just coffee. Do not use propranolol in situations where you may need extra adrenaline, such as athletic events or other activities requiring great physical exertion. Propranolol should not be used by people with asthma or arterial spasms. Propranolol should not be used by people within two weeks of having taken an MAO inhibitor or certain other drugs for psychiatric problems (check with your doctor) or during the pollen season, if you suffer from pollen allergies. Use with caution if you have chronic bronchitis or emphysema. If you are diabetic, you should be watched carefully by your doctor. Use cautiously if you have kidney or liver problems. The safe use of propranolol during pregnancy has not been established.

Dosage: 10 to 30mg one and a half hours before the event that usually causes a fear response. Propranolol can cause nausea if taken on an empty stomach, especially if it is taken with coffee and no food.

Sources: Propranolol is available in the U.S.A. with a doctor's prescription. Keep in mind, however, that your doctor may not be familiar with the uses we have discussed. Propranolol can also be purchased over the counter in Mexico or by mail order from the sources listed in Appendix A (see page 165). Other names for propranolol include: Angilol, Apsolol, Avlocardyl, Bedranol, Beprane, Berkolol, Beta-Neg, Beta-Tablinen, Beta-Timelets, Cardinol, Caridorol, Deralin, Dociton, Dumopranol, Duranol, Efektolol, Elbrol, Euprovasin, Frekven, Inderal, Inderex, Indobloc, Intermigran, Kemi, Oposim, Prano-Puren, Propahexal, Prophylux, Propranur, Pylapron, Rapynogen, Sagittol, Sloprolol, Sumial, and Tesnol.

References:

Brantigan, C.O., Brantigen, T.A., Joseph, N. "The Effect of Beta Blockade on Stage Fright. A Controlled Study." **Rocky Mountain Medical Journal.** Sep-Oct 1979, 76 (5) pp. 227-33.

Foster, G.E., Evans, D.F., Hardcastle, J.D. "Heart-Rates of Surgeons During Operations and Other Clinical Activities and Their Modification by Oxprenolol." **The Lancet.** June 24, 1978, pp. 1323-5.

Liden, S., Gottfries, C., "Beta-Blocking Agents in the Treatment of Catecholamine-Induced Symptoms in Musicians." **The Lancet.** August 31, 1974, p. 529.

Mason, D., Dyller, F. **Pharmaceutical Dictionary & Reference** New York: Playboy Paperbacks, 1982.

James, I.M., Pearson, R.M., Griffith, D.N.W., Newbury, P. "Effect of Oxprenolol on Stage-Fright in Musicians." **The Lancet.** November 5, 1977, pp. 952-4.

Pearson, D., Shaw, S. **Life Extension: A Practical Scientific Approach**. New York: Warner Books, 1982.

Thyroid Hormone

One cause of poor concentration ability, mental confusion, and memory disturbances that is frequently overlooked by doctors is borderline inadequate thyroid function. Physicians call this condition subclinical hypothyroidism. Subclinical hypothyroidism is frequently accompanied by a spectrum of symptoms that include (in addition to mental dysfunction): cold hands and feet, menstrual problems, dry skin, thin hair, and low energy levels. In his book, *Hypothyroidism: The Unsuspected Illness*, Dr. Broda Barnes described over 47 symptoms that may be related to poor thyroid function.

Dr. Barnes developed a simple test to confirm suspected low thyroid function using an ordinary thermometer. He found that in the absence of oral infection, the temperatures of the mouth and the armpit were identical when the thermometers were left in place for 10 minutes. He found that normal values for temperatures immediately upon wakening in the morning (while still in bed) are in the range of 97.8 to 98.2 degrees Fahrenheit. A temperature below 97.8 indicates hypothyroidism, one above 98.2, hyperthyroidism (overactive thyroid). Because of his finding that the oral and armpit temperatures were identical, he inexplicably recommended the underarm temperature taken immediately upon awakening be used exclusively to diagnose borderline hypothyroidism. It is clear that the oral temperature taken at the same time serves exactly the same purpose. One of the co-authors

(Ward Dean, M.D.) advises his patients to avoid the "ritual" of the underarm measurement and use the standard oral temperature taken immediately upon awakening in the morning as a guide to diagnosis and treatment of hypothyroidism.

Precautions: Thyroid drugs should only be used under a physician's supervision. Names of physicians who are generally familiar with Barnes' method of diagnosis and treatment can be obtained from the American College of Advancement in Medicine, (714) 583 7666 or (800) 532 3688.

Treatment of subclinical hypothyroidism with thyroid hormone is very safe. To avoid overdose, the resting pulse rate should be recorded each time the temperature is taken. Normal resting pulse should be less than 72 beats per minute. As long as the temperature remains below 98.2, the pulse is less than 72 beats per minute, and thyroid function tests remain normal, there is little risk of excessive thyroid dosage (Barnes, 1976). Although several recent studies indicate that synthetic thyroid hormone (1-thyroxine) may cause bone loss (Coindre, 1986; Kung, 1991), bone loss has never been demonstrated with the natural form of thyroid that is generally prescribed by physicians who adhere to the Barnes protocol.

References:

Barnes, B., Galton, L. **Hypothyroidism: the Unsuspected Illness.** New York: Thomas Y. Crowell Co., 1976.
Coindre, J.M., David, J.P., Riviere, L., et al. "Bone Loss in Hypo-

thyroidism with Hormone Replacement: A Histomorphometric Study." **Archives of Internal Medicine.** 1986, 146, pp. 48-53.

Kung, A.W.C., Pun, K.K. "Bone Mineral Density in Premenopausal Women Receiving Long-Term Physiological Doses of Levo-thyroxine." **Journal of the American Medical Association.** 1991, 265, 20, pp. 2688-91.

Langer, S., Scheer, J. **Solved: the Riddle of Illness.** New Canaan, CT: Keats, 1984.

Vasopressin (Diapid)

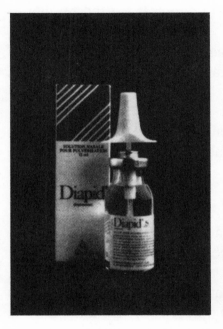

Vasopressin (anti-diuretic hormone) is a hormone secreted by the posterior portion of the pituitary gland. It is approved for treatment of diabetes insipidus because it prevents the frequent urination that occurs in this disease. Vasopressin has also been used to treat memory deficits due to aging, senile dementia, Alzheimer's disease, Korsakoff's Syndrome and amnesia. It improves attention, concentration, memory retention, and recall (both short-term and long-term). Vasopressin is necessary for imprinting new information in your memory.

Cocaine, LSD, amphetamines, Ritalin, and Cylert (pemoline) cause your pituitary gland to release natural vasopressin at a faster rate. Frequent use of these drugs can cause depleted levels of vasopressin with resultant slowness and dopiness. A whiff of vasopressin can transform stimulant burnout experience in about 10 seconds, because it is rapidly ab-

143

sorbed by the nasal mucosa, and immediately replaces the vasopressin that has been depleted.

Conversely, marijuana and alcohol suppress the release of vasopressin. A whiff of vasopressin when using these drugs will compensate for much of the dopiness caused by them.

Vasopressin is very useful when learning large amounts of new information. It can increase your ability to memorize and recall.

Many people have very strong and positive reactions to vasopressin. We include a number of testimonials in Appendix D (see page 179).

Precautions: Vasopressin occasionally produces the following side effects: nasal congestion, runny nose, itch or irritation of the nasal passages, abdominal cramps, headache, and increased bowel movements. Vasopressin has not been proven to be safe for use during pregnancy. It should also be used cautiously in cases of hypertension or epilepsy.

Dosage: Vasopressin usually comes in a nasal spray bottle. Most studies showing memory improvement have been done with a dose of 12 to 16 USP units per day, or about two whiffs three or four times per day. Vasopressin produces a noticeable effect within seconds.

Sources: Vasopressin is available in the U.S.A. You can buy it with a doctor's prescription. Again, keep in mind that most physicians may not be familiar with the uses we discuss here. It can also be purchased over the counter in Mexico or by mail order from the sources listed in Appendix A (see page

165).

Vasopressin comes in three forms: lysine-vasopressin (Diapid, LVP, Lypressin, Postacton, Syntopressin), 1-desamino-8-D-arginine (Adiuretin SD, DAV Ritter, DDAVP, Desmopressin, Desmospray, Minirin), and arginine-vasopressin (argipressin, AVP, rinder-vasopressin). All forms have very similar or identical effects.

References:

de Wied, D., van Wimersma Greidanus, T.B., Bohus, B., Urban, I., Gispen, W.H. "Vasopressin and Memory Consolidation." **Perspectives in Brain Research**. New York: Elsevier Scientific Publishing, 1975.

Gold, P.W., Weingartner, H., Ballenger, J.C., Goodwin, F.K., Post, R.M. "Effects of 1-Desamo-8-Arginine Vasopressin on Behavior and Cognition in Primary Affective Disorders." **The Lancet**. November 10, 1979, pp. 992-94.

Laczi, F., Valkusz, Z., Laszlo, F.A., Wagner, A., Jardanhazy, T., Szasz, A., Szilard, J., Telegdy, G. "Effects of Lysine-Vasopressin and 1-Deamino-8-D-Arginine-Vasopressin on Memory in Healthy Individuals and Diabetes Insipidus Patients." **Psychoneuroendocrinology**. 1982, Vol. 7, No. 2, pp. 185-92.

Legros, J.J., Gilot, P., Seron, X., Claessens, J., Adam, A., Moeglen, J.M., Audibert, A., Berchier, P. "Influence of Vasopressin on Learning and Memory." **The Lancet**. January 7, 1978, pp. 41-42.

Oliveros, J.C., Jandali, M.K., Timsit-Berthier, M., Remy, R., Benghezal, A., Audibert, A., Moeglen, J.M. "Vasopressin in Amnesia." **The Lancet**. January 7, 1978, p. 42.

Pearson, D., Shaw, S. **Life Extension: A Practical Scientific Approach**. New York: Warner Books, 1982.

Pelton, R., Pelton, T.C. **Mind Food & Smart Pills**. New York: Doubleday, 1989.

Vincamine

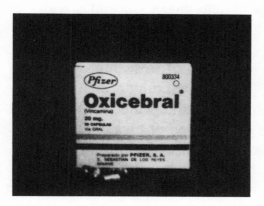

Vincamine is an extract of the periwinkle. It is a vasodilator and increases blood flow to the brain and improves the brain's use of oxygen.

Vincamine has been used to treat a remarkable variety of conditions related to insufficient blood flow to the brain, including vertigo and Meniere's syndrome, difficulty in sleeping, mood changes, depression, hearing problems, high blood pressure and lack of blood flow to the eyes. Vincamine has also been used for improving memory defects and inability to concentrate. Vincamine has extremely low toxicity and is very inexpensive.

Vincamine has shown some efficacy in the treatment of Alzheimer's disease (Albert, 1983, Branconnier, 1983). Vincamine normalizes the brain-wave patterns of elderly people with bad memories and alcohol-induced organic brain syndrome (Moglia, 1984, Saletu, 1985).

If you have a family member or friend who is suffering from some form of senility, talk to their physician about vincamine. Its low cost and low toxicity make vincamine a logical choice to be included in a combination drug therapy.

We have not found a great deal of research involving vincamine and cognitive enhancement in normal, healthy humans. We do know that people like vincamine. People report that the subjective effects are very pleasant, and that it seems to enhance memory and concentration.

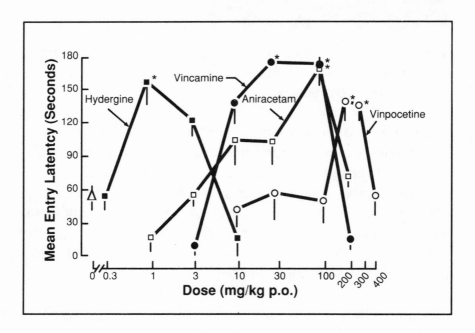

In this study, inexpensive vincamine compares favorably with other cognition enhancers in protecting rats from scopolamine-induced memory impairment. (Redrawn from DeNoble, 1986.)

Precautions: Rarely causes gastrointestinal distress, which disappears when usage is stopped. Vincamine has not been proven to be safe for pregnant women or children.

Dosage: 30mg every 12 hours.

Sources: Vincamine can be purchased in Europe or by mail order from the sources listed in Appendix A (see page 165). Other names include: Aethroma, Anasclerol, Angiopac, Arteriovinca, Asnai, Cerebroxine, Cetal, Cetovinca, Cincuental, Devincan, Equipur, Esberidin, Novicet, Ocu-Vinc, Oxicebral, Oxygeron, Perval, Pervincamin, Pervone, Sostenil, Tripervan, Venoxigen, Vinca, Vincabiomar, Vincabrain, Vincadar, Vincafarm, Vincafolina, Vincafor, Vincagil, Vincahexal, Vincalen, Vincamidol, Vincane, Vincapan, Vincapront, Vincasaunier, Vincavix, Vincimax, Vinodrel Retard, Vinodrel, and Vraap.

References:

Albert, M. "Treating Memory Disorders in the Elderly." **Drug Therapy**. October, 1983, pp. 257-65.

Anderson, K., Anderson, L. **Orphan Drugs**. Los Angeles, CA: The Body Press, 1987.

Branconnier, R. "The Efficacy of the Cerebral Metabolic Enhancers in the Treatment of Senile Dementia." **Psychopharmacology Bulletin**. 1983, 19(2), pp. 212-20.

Casale, R., Giorgi, I., Guarnaschelli, C. "Evaluation of the Effect of Vincamine Teprosilate on Behavioral Performances of Patients Affected with Chronic Cerebrovascular Disease." **International Journal of Clinical Pharmacology Research**. 1984, 4 (4) pp. 313-9.

DeNoble, V.J., Repetti, S.J., Gelpke, L.W., Wood, L.M., Keim, K.L. "Vinpocetine: Nootropic Effects on Scopolamine-Induced and Hypoxia-Induced Retrieval Deficits of a Step-Through Passive

Avoidance Response in Rats." **Pharmacology Biochemistry & Behavior.** 1986, Vol. 24, pp. 1123-8.

Groo, D., Palosi, E., Szporny, L. "Comparison of the Effects of Vinpocetine, Vincamine, and Nicergoline on the Normal and Hypoxia Damaged Learning Process in Spontaneously Hypertensive Rats." **Drug Development Research.** 1988, 15: pp. 75-85.

Moglia, A., Alfonsi, E., Zandrini, C., Pistarini, C., Arrigo, A. "Acute I.V. Vincamine Teprosilate Administration: Quantified Investigation in Elderly Subjects. **International Journal of Clinical Pharmacology Research.** 1984, 4 (4) pp. 303-6.

Novis, S.P., Moretto, M., Fenelon, S.B., Barbosa, C.S., da Graca Torres, J. "Vincamine in Patients with Cerebral Vascular Insufficiency" **Arquivos Neuropsiquiatria.** 1975, 33 (1) pp. 25-32.

Saletu, B., Grunberger, J. "Memory Dysfunction and Vigilance: Neurophysiological and Psychopharmacological Aspects." **Annals of the New York Academy of Sciences.** 1985, Vol. 444, pp. 406-27.

Vitamins

Vitamins are substances that are essential to life. All of the biochemical reactions in our bodies rely on vitamins in some way. Some vitamins delay aging-related intelligence decline and improve intelligence and reaction time. We include in this section a few examples of the relationship between vitamins and intelligence. For more information, please refer to the resources we list in Appendix E (see page 185). Sources for vitamins are listed in Appendix A (see page 165).

A survey of 37,875 Americans found that 80% of the subjects consumed less than the Recommended Daily Allowances (RDAs) of at least one vitamin each day (Pao, 1981).

Choline, in all its different forms, is often referred to as a vitamin. We have accorded choline its own section in this book due to its value as an intelligence-enhancing and memory-enhancing agent.

Antioxidants

Many of the vitamins and some of the other substances in this book, such as Hydergine, are antioxidants. This means that they prevent uncontrolled oxidization of molecules in our bodies. Uncontrolled oxidization is caused by free radicals that are generated by ultra-violet rays from the sun, certain foods that we eat, cigarettes and other drugs, and even natural biological processes. Oxidization can create a number of different problems in our brains and nervous systems.

One example is alcohol-induced oxidization. Alcoholics often have wrinkles and leathery skin caused by the oxidization of collagen and other important molecules in the skin. Likewise, alcoholics are prone to Korsakoff's syndrome, a condition similar to senility. Korsakoff's is caused by overindulgence in alcohol and a lack of vitamin B-1, a powerful antioxidant.

For excellent treatments of the subject of antioxidants and aging, see Pearson and Shaw's *Life Extension*, Linus Pauling's *How to Live Longer and Feel Better*, Sheldon Saul Hendler's *Complete Guide To Anti-Aging Nutrients*, and Lord Lee-Benner's *Physician's Guide to Free Radicals, Immunity, and Aging* listed in the references below and reviewed in Appendix E on page 185.

B Vitamins

B vitamins are necessary for the health of your nervous system, for proper mental functioning, and many other processes. Because of their many uses, we have included individual descriptions of five B vitamins. However, the B vitamins are an interlocking complex. Thus, even if you are most interested in the role that one of them plays, you should be sure that you are getting others in the complex by including a B-complex, or a multiple with B-complex, in your daily regimen.

B vitamins exert a great influence on fine motor control. One double-blind placebo-controlled study found that normal, healthy volunteers who were experienced marksmen improved their aim significantly by taking a vitamin B formulation containing vitamins B-1, B-6, and B-12. (Bonke, 1986).

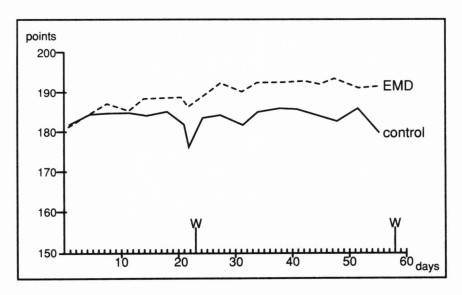

Improvement in shooting accuracy in normal, healthy subjects given a B vitamin complex with B-1, B-6, and B-12 (EMD) versus a placebo. "W" marks a competition day. (Redrawn from Bonke, 1986.)

B vitamins, like vitamin C, are water soluble in your body. This means that they are not stored in your fat cells. If you take them, divide the dose into three or four parts and take them with each meal.

Vitamin B-1

B-1, or thiamine, is a powerful antioxidant. As mentioned previously, B-1 can protect your nerve tissues against the oxidizing effects of alcohol, but it also protects against many other oxidizing agents. Many of the studies we cite in this book refer to the treatment of organic brain syndrome, much of which is caused by long-term alcohol abuse.

Dosage: 50mg-1000mg per day. Best taken in 3 or 4 divided doses with meals.

Vitamin B-3 (Niacin)

Niacin, also called vitamin B-3, has many interesting health benefits including memory enhancement. In one study, 141mg of niacin per day improved memory in both young and middle-aged normal, healthy subjects by 10-40% (Loriaux, 1985). The study was conducted as a double-blind placebo-controlled study.

Precautions: If you have diabetes, high blood pressure, ulcers or porphyria, niacin should be taken under the supervision of a physician experienced in vitamin therapy. Niacin is very acidic. People with ulcers may need to take an antacid such as bicarbonate of soda (avoid antacids containing aluminum) with niacin. Some people experience a skin flush or redness and tingling, dizziness or headache for 10 or 20 minutes when first taking niacin. Flushing is much more likely to occur if the niacin is taken on an empty stomach. The flushing is not harmful, and should disappear after niacin is taken for several weeks or so.

Dosage: Most people start off at low doses of niacin (not niacinamide) and gradually build up to 100 to 200mg per day

(For cholesterol-lowering effects, the dosage is usually 10 times this much). The dosage should be divided into 3 or 4 doses and taken with meals. Some people may get a niacin flush with this dose. With continued daily use, you will develop a tolerance for the flush.

Vitamin B-5

B-5, or pantothenic acid, has many functions in the body, including being a powerful antioxidant and stamina enhancer. B-5 is essential for the formation of steroid hormones, making it particularly important for individuals under stress, since such persons secrete more adrenal cortex hormones than others (Newbold, 1975). Note that B-5 is essential for the conversion of choline into acetylcholine.

Precautions: Large dosages may at first cause diarrhea. This effect disappears with continued use.

Dosage: Most people start out at 100mg and slowly work up to 250mg-1000mg per day in 3 or 4 divided doses with meals.

Vitamin B-6

Vitamin B-6, or pyridoxine, is necessary for the manufacture of many neurotransmitters. Without sufficient B-6, your body may not produce enough norepinephrine, serotonin or dopamine. These neurotransmitters are essential to optimum mental functioning. Since B-6 is used in protein metabolism, a high-protein diet often causes an elevated need for B-6

(Newbold, 1975).

Precautions: People using the drug L-Dopa for the treatment of Parkinson's disease should not take vitamin B-6 except under the supervision of a physician. Dosages greater than 200mg per day have caused peripheral neuropathy and should never be taken without the recommendation of a physician.

Dosage: 50mg-200mg per day in 3 or 4 divided doses.

Vitamin B-12

B-12, or cyanocobalamin, stimulates RNA synthesis in nerve cells and increases the rate of learning in lab rats. (Pearson and Shaw, 1982). Many vegetarians do not get enough B-12 in their diets. The drug Dilantin may cause a marked depletion of B-12. Low thyroid can reduce B-12 absorption.

Precautions: People with gout should use B-12 only with extreme caution.

Dosage: 1mg (1000 micrograms) per day. Since some people have difficulty absorbing B-12 orally, it is also available in sublingual form as well as in a nasal applicator. It can also be given by injection by your doctor.

Vitamin C

Vitamin C, also called ascorbic acid, is a key antioxidant in our bodies, and is necessary for the manufacture of neurotransmitters and cell (including nerve cell) structures.

Precautions: If too much vitamin C is taken gas and diarrhea can result. This effect disappears when the dosage is reduced.

Dosage: 2000-5000mg per day in 3 or 4 divided doses.

Vitamin E

Vitamin E is a powerful fat-soluble antioxidant. This may be its only function in our cells. By preventing the oxidation of important molecules in our cells, vitamin E may retard the aging process. Vitamin E is found in high concentration in the lipid fraction of cell membranes. This is where prostaglandins are synthesized. Prostaglandins are extremely fast acting hormones that mediate all biological processes, including thought. The oils from which prostaglandins are synthesized, and the prostaglandins themselves, are extremely susceptible to oxidation, hence the high concentrations of protective vitamin E in the cell membranes.

Precautions: Vitamin E has no known toxicity. People with heart disease or high blood pressure should start at low dosages and only with a doctors supervision. This is because vitamin E can cause a rise in blood pressure when it is first taken.

Dosage: 100-1000 I.U. per day.

Dosage For Vitamins

The "recommended daily allowances", or RDAs, of the vitamins were originally formulated by measuring the quantity of each vitamin Americans normally consumed. Due to the difficulty and expense of establishing the optimum dose of each vitamin for humans, the RDAs are actually a statement of how much of each vitamin a human needs in order to avoid vitamin deficiency diseases like scurvy. As we mentioned in the introduction to this section, a recent survey of the eating habits of 37,785 Americans established that 80% consumed less than the RDA of at least one vitamin (Pao, 1979).

There is much research which indicates that doses much higher than the RDAs have many beneficial effects. By dividing the dose of the water-soluble vitamins, you will assure that your cells have the vitamins they need all day long.

References:

Bonke, D. "Influence of vitamin B-1, B-6, B-12 on the Control of Fine Motor Movement." **Bibliotheca Nutritio et Dieta**. 1986, 38, pp. 104-9.

Hendler, S.S. **The Complete Guide To Anti-Aging Nutrients**. New York: Simon & Schuster, 1985.

Lee-Benner, L. **Physician's Guide to Free Radicals, Immunity, and Aging**. Newport Beach: World Health Foundation, 1991.

Loriaux, S.M., Deijen, J.B., Orlebeke, J.F., De Swart, J.H. "The Effects of Nicotinic Acid (Niacin) and Xanthinol Nicotinate on Human Memory in Different Categories of Age, a Double Blind Study." **Psychopharmacology**. 1985, Vol. 87, pp. 390-395.

Newbold, H.L. **Meganutrients for Your Nerves**. New York: Berkeley Books, 1975.

Pao, E., Mickle, S. "Problem Nutrients in the United States." **Food Technology**. September, 1981. pp. 58-69, 79.

Pauling, L. **How to Live Longer and Feel Better**. New York: W. H. Freeman, 1986.

Pearson, D., Shaw, S. **Life Extension: A Practical Scientific Approach**. New York: Warner Books, 1982.

Pelton, R., Pelton, T.C. **Mind Food & Smart Pills**. New York: Doubleday, 1989.

Xanthinol Nicotinate

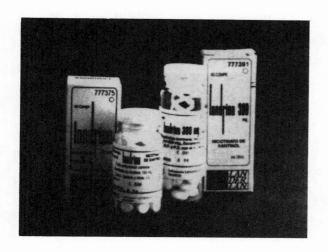

Xanthinol nicotinate is a form of niacin that can pass easily through the cell membrane into the cell much more readily than niacin. Once inside the cell, xanthinol nicotinate causes an increase in glucose metabolism and a corresponding increase in ATP, the universal energy molecule.

Xanthinol nicotinate is a vasodilator and is used as an agent to lower serum cholesterol. The drug has been used to treat insufficient blood flow to the brain, arteries, and the extremities (Anderson, 1987).

A double-blind placebo-controlled study was conducted comparing 500mg of xanthinol nicotinate with 141.7mg of niacin (500mg of xanthinol nicotinate contains 141.7mg of niacin chemically bonded to xanthinol). Xanthinol nicotinate was found to improve performance of normal, healthy elderly people on a variety of short-term and long-term memory tests (Loriaux, 1985). We previously cited the study by Loriaux in the section on niacin. It shows the remarkable short-term memory improvements in young and middle aged people using niacin. Xanthinol nicotinate also significantly improved reaction times in the elderly subjects of this study.

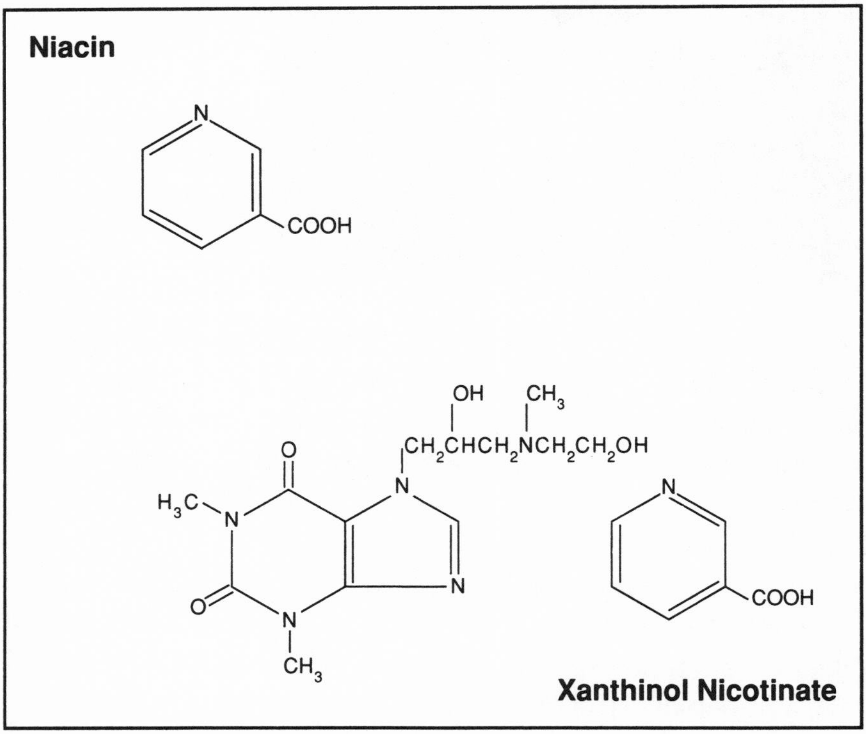

Niacin

Xanthinol Nicotinate

Precautions: Xanthinol Nicotinate may cause flushing or a sense of warmth. It can also cause heart palpitations, nausea, vomiting, heartburn, diarrhea, headache, muscle cramps, or blurred vision. These effects often disappear with continued usage. Some people may experience itchy skin, rash, or changes in skin color. Xanthinol Nicotinate may cause postural hypotension (a drop in blood pressure when standing up from a sitting position) because of its vasodilation effect. Safety in pregnant women and nursing mothers has not been established. Xanthinol nicotinate should not be used by people with peptic ulcers, congestive heart failure, severe hypotension, or liver problems or by people who have had a recent myocardial infarction.

Dosage: 900 - 1800mg per day in divided doses taken with meals. Maximum dosage is 3000mg.

Sources: Xanthinol nicotinate can be purchased in Europe or Canada or by mail order from the sources listed in Appendix A (see page 165). Other names include: Androgeron, Angiomanin, Angiomin, Cafardil, Circulan, Clofamin, Complamex, Complamin, Dacilin, Emodinamin, Jupal, Landrina, Niconicol, Sadamin, SK 331 A, Vasoprin, Vedrin, Xanidil, Xavin, and Xavin.

References:

Anderson, K., Anderson, L. **Orphan Drugs**. Los Angeles, CA: The Body Press, 1987.
Loriaux, S.M., Deijen, J.B., Orlebeke, J.F., De Swart, J.H. "The Effects of Nicotinic Acid (Niacin) and Xanthinol Nicotinate on Human Memory in Different Categories of Age, a Double Blind Study." **Psychopharmacology**. 1985, Vol. 87, pp. 390-395.

Appendix A: Product Sources

In the first printing of this book we listed several overseas mail-order sources for smart drugs and nutrients. Since then, the state of availability of smart drugs has entered a period of change. Some of the original sources we listed have gone out of business, and others have changed their addresses. The FDA policy toward some smart drugs seems to be in a state of flux. Additionally, we have discovered new sources.

Due to the changes, we have decided not to list any overseas mail-order sources here since they could change shortly after printing. Please write to CERI (the Cognitive Enhancement Research Institute) and request their Smart Drug Sources List.

> Cognition Enhancement Research Institute
> POB 4029-2009
> Menlo Park, CA 94026-4029

Please include $2.00 for postage and handling. CERI's list is updated on a monthly basis. You can get the latest information on which sources are most reliable and least expensive.

We also strongly encourage you to subscribe to CERI's newsletter, **Smart Drug News**. The price is $40 per year for 10 issues. The list of smart drug sources mentioned above is provided free to subscribers. **Smart Drug News** covers the latest smart drug and nutrient research. In the question and answer section, subscribers can get their questions answered by experts on smart drugs.

Smart drugs are available in many foreign countries. Pharmacies in Mexico, for example, often stock most of the drugs listed in this book. U.S. Customs has traditionally allowed personal importation of foreign drugs for personal use. Some people have told us that they combine their vacation plans with buying trips. Other countries where readers have reported purchasing smart drugs include: Thailand, Italy, Spain, and Belgium.

In this appendix, we include a few of the most reliable sources for smart nutrients in the United States. These sources cannot sell drugs such as piracetam and hydergine.

Smart Nutrients By Mail

Life Services Supplements, Inc.
81 First Ave., Dept. 13
Atlantic Highlands, NJ 07716
Phone: (800) 542 3230 or (201) 872 8700

Life Services is a mail order company and world-wide licensee to market and manufacture all 28 Durk Pearson and Sandy Shaw Designer Food™ formulations. All ingredients are purchased from high quality sources. Life Services guarantees same day shipping on all orders received prior to 4 PM ET. They also will conduct searches for you of computer data-bases such as Med-Line, the database of the National Library of Medicine.

NutriGuard Research
P.O. Box 865-A
Encinitas, CA 92023
Phone: (800) 433 2402 or (619) 942 3223

NutriGuard sells a comprehensive line of high-quality nutritional supplements that includes vitamins, minerals, amino acids, and essential fatty acids. The products are available in capsules, tablets, and powders. NutriGuard generally has low prices—they have the lowest price we have seen for 50% phosphatidyl choline. Technical data sheets are available which describe the rationale for the formulations.

Responsible Health, Inc.
3535 E. Coast Highway, Suite 231-C
Corona Del Mar, CA 92625
Phone: (714) 720 9110

Responsible Health manufactures a line of nutritional supplements based on the concepts in Dr. Lord Lee-Benner's book, *Physician's Guide to Free Radicals, Immunity and Aging.*

Smart Products
870 Market Street, Suite 1262-SD
San Francisco, CA 94102
Phone: (800) 858 6520 or (415) 989 2500

Smart Products offers a free newsletter, books, videos and the complete line of Pearson & Shaw products.

Smart Buys At Health & Vitamin Stores

Health-food and vitamin stores offer a wide variety of smart nutrients. Many stores offer high-quality products from these two nutrient manufacturers.

Source Naturals
P.O. Box 2118
Santa Cruz, CA 95063
Phone: (408) 438 6851

TwinLab
Ronkonkoma, NY 11779
Phone: (516) 467 3140

Source Naturals has created the Body/Mind Series. These products are specifically designed for cognitive enhancement. They are available in many health food and vitamin stores or can be ordered by a store for you. Source Naturals offers innovative formulas including choline, lecithin, DMAE, Ginkgo biloba extract, ginseng, EggsACT brand AL721, PCA, and vitamins. Nearly all the products are vegetarian tablets with the lowest possible amounts of excipients and binders.

TwinLab is the manufacturer of a complete line of nutritional products in capsules. Their products are available in most health food and vitamin stores. Their quality is uniformly excellent.

More Smart Drug & Nutrient Sources

PWA Health Group
31 W. 26th St. 4th Fl.
New York, NY 10010
Phone: (212) 532 0363

PWA Health Group is a not-for-profit organization formed to supply people with AIDS with hard-to-get AIDS treatments. They carry some smart drugs and nutrients such as AL721 and DHEA.

Compounding Pharmacists

College Pharmacy
Phone: (800) 888 9358

College Pharmacy of Colorado Springs, Colorado specializes in custom environmental compounding. Hard to find preparations are their specialty. Doctors can contact them by calling their toll-free number.

Appendix B:
Aluminum and Alzheimer's Disease

When people with Alzheimer's disease die and their brains are examined, researchers usually find aluminum ions. Aluminum is a highly reactive cross-linking agent. Such an agent binds separate molecules or parts of the same molecule. Molecules thus bound are no longer able to absorb water, oxygen, or nutrients from the blood vessels (Kaufman 1986). Aluminum is used to tan the covers of baseballs because it cross-links and hardens the leather.

When injected into the brains of experimental animals, aluminum causes neurofibrillary tangles (tangles of nerve filaments). These tangles are also found in the brains of people with Alzheimer's disease.

Aluminum can reduce the transport of choline into nerve cells. Choline is the precursor of acetylcholine, a neurotransmitter (see choline). People with Alzheimer's disease have low levels of acetylcholine in their brains.

Aluminum sulfate is used by water utilities to remove fine particles from drinking water. One recent study found that areas in England that had elevated levels of aluminum sulfate in the drinking water have elevated incidence of Alzheimer's disease (Martyn, 1989).

Whether aluminum is the actual cause of Alzheimer's disease is still a matter of scientific controversy. It is, however, classified as a toxic metal, and many people will wish to minimize their intake of aluminum. Here too, there is controversy. Aluminum cookware is totally avoided by some, while others only avoid it for the cooking of acid foods. Everyone involved with this issue should be aware that aluminum is also found in less obvious places: deodorants, antacids and baking powder. As for drinking water, we have listed information below about a water filter for removing aluminum sulfate from drinking water.

More reasons for concern about aluminum are brewing. Researchers recently have begun developing data that suggests that aluminum also may be linked to multiple sclerosis and Parkinson's disease (Piccardo, 1988).

Two fruit acids, citric acid and malic acid, have been demonstrated to facilitate the excretion of aluminum in mouse experiments. The acids are commonly found in foods such as fruit and wine, and are used as flavorings. Citric acid and malic acid bond with the aluminum and carry it out of the body safely. Malic acid is better than citric at removing aluminum from brain and nerve tissue and citric acid is better at removing aluminum from body tissue of lab mice.

Durk Pearson and Sandy Shaw report hearing of a very strange case where one identical twin sister had come down with Alzheimer's disease while after 10 years the other twin had not. The researcher describing the case told Pearson and Shaw that the twins both ate the same food and drank the same water. The researcher found only one difference in the two women's lifestyles—the woman who did not get Alzheimer's disease had been drinking half a bottle of wine per day for years. Pearson and Shaw note that half of a bottle of wine contains about 1.5 grams of malic acid. This story is not proof of anything in the scientific sense, but it raises questions for further research.

When we discuss a smart drug or nutrient in this book, we usually do so because we find a large body of research establishing its efficacy. In this case there are only a few papers showing that fruit acids remove aluminum from the brain and body. Also, we have not seen any studies that tried to show the effectiveness of these fruit acids in treating or preventing Alzheimer's disease.

Having said this, we nevertheless included the information about fruit acids in this appendix for two reasons. First, we hope that this might stimulate some well-planned scientific research into the potential of fruit acids. Second, we realize that many people will be willing to try a common substance of low cost and apparent lack of side effects without waiting for scientific validation. If you do plan to add fruit acids to the diet of an Alzheimer's patient, inform the physician involved.

Sources for fruit acids: Fruit acids are found in significant quantities in wine, apples, cherries, and other fruits. We would not, of course, recommend drinking half a bottle of wine per day. Fruit acids are also included as flavoring agents in many soda pop drinks, but we have no data on the quantities used. Pearson and Shaw have developed a number of nutrient drink formulas that contain fruit acids as flavoring agents where the quantity is known. One example is a choline drink formula that contains 1.8 grams of citric acid and 200mg of malic acid per serving. See Appendix A (page 165) to find out where to purchase these drink mixes.

We would like anyone who uses fruit acids or the Pearson and Shaw drink mixes for the treatment of Alzheimer's disease to contact us. Any data we collect can serve as a direction for future research.

Precautions: Some persons who have herpes simplex get cold sores when they increase their fruit acid intake. Others are allergic to citrus. We do not know of any other adverse effects of citric or malic acid.

Sources for a water filter for filtering aluminum: We have seen a chemical analysis of water filtered through a Multi-Pure Model 500 Activated Carbon Block water filter that indicates that the filter removes more than 99.99% of aluminum sulfate from the water. Multi-Pure filters can be purchased from:

Multi-Pure Drinking Water Systems
P.O. Box 8190
Santa Cruz, CA 95061

Write for a free brochure and a copy of the aluminum sulfate assay.

Other water filters may remove aluminum sulfate, but be certain that the manufacturer has tested the filter for filtering aluminum and can show you a test assay.

References:

Domingo, J., et al. "Citric, Malic and Succinic Acids as Possible Alternatives to Deferoxamine in Aluminum Toxicity." **Journal of Toxicology - Clinical Toxicology.** 1988, 26 (1-2), pp. 67-79.

Kaufman, R. **The Age Reduction System**. New York: Rawson Associates 1986.

Martyn, C.N., Barker, D.J.P., Osmond, C., Harris, F.C., Edwardson, J.A., Lacey, R.F. "Geographical Relation Between Alzheimer's Disease and Aluminum in Drinking Water." **The Lancet**. January 14, 1989, pp. 59-62.

Pearson, D., Shaw, S. Durk **Pearson & Sandy Shaw's Life Extension Newsletter**. June 1988, Vol 1, Number 4, p. 30.

Pearson, D., Shaw, S. Durk **Pearson & Sandy Shaw's Life Extension Newsletter**. November 1988, Vol 1, Number 9, p. 74. Ibid. January 1989, Vol 1, Number 11, p. 98.

Pearson, D., Shaw, S. Durk **Pearson & Sandy Shaw's Life Extension Newsletter**. January-February 1990, Vol 2, Number 10, pp. 84-6.

Piccardo, P., Yanagihara, R., Garruto, R.M., Gibbs, C.J. Jr., Gajdusek, D.C. "Histochemical and X-ray Microanalytical Localization of Aluminum in Amyotrophic Lateral Sclerosis and Parkinsonism-Dementia of Guam." **Acta Neuropathologica**. 1988, 77 (1) pp.1-4.

Appendix C:
Other Smart Drugs & Nutrients

Here is a list of smart drugs and nutrients, safe and unsafe, that are not discussed in this book. We devoted full sections to the compounds we thought are most interesting and which also met our criteria: data showing efficacy, low side effects, etc. If there is a lot of reader interest in particular items listed here, and they meet our criteria, they will be covered in a future edition of this book or a newsletter.

If you have relevant data to share about the cognitive-enhancement properties of any of these substances, please write to B&J Publications, P.O. Box 2515-HC, Menlo Park, CA 94026.

3-4 DAP
aceglutamide
ACTH 4-10
ACTH 4-9 (analog)
adafenoxate
almitrine
amphetamines
arecoline
beta-carbolines
cayenne

chlorpromazine
CI-844
CI-911
CI-933
cinnarizine
citicoline
cyclandelate
deprenyl
DGLVP
dihydroergocryptine

dupracetam
ebiratide (Hoe 427)
eburnamonine
edrophonium
EMD 21657
ergot derivatives
etiracetam
flunarizine
fluoxetine
glutamine
glutaurine   (gamma-L-glu-
    tamyl-taurine)
glycosaminoglycan polysul-
    phate
GM-1
gotu kola
guanfacine
HOE 175
HR 001
imipramine
L-prolyl L-leucyl   glycine
    amide
lergotrile
lithium chloride
metrazole
MK 771
naftidrofuryl
naloxone
neuropeptides
nicergoline
nicotine
nimodipine
oxotremorine
oxpentifylline

parlodel
pemoline
pentoxifylline
phenobarbital
phosphatidylserine
physostigmine
picrotoxin
polygala
PRL-8-53
pyritinol
R-58-735 (Sabeluzole)
Ritalin
RNA (ribonucleic acid)
rolziracetam
schizandra
somatostatin
sulbutiamine
tenilsetam
tranylcypromine
TRH
UCB LO59
valproate
zarontin
zimeldine

Appendix D:
Testimonials & Case Histories

Testimonials and case histories are always suspect in scientific circles. This is because the human mind is so powerful at producing the placebo effect. Humans repeatedly experience powerful drug effects from taking inactive substances when they believe that the substances are drugs. That is why we rely on references to scientific research for the information we present.

We include this appendix of testimonials and case histories so that you may orient yourself as to which smart drugs and nutrients you might like to try. If you would like to share your experiences with us, whether they are similar or different than the ones described here, please feel free to write to the authors c/o B&J Publications, P.O. Box 2515-HC, Menlo Park, CA 94026.

Piracetam:

"My secretary responded so well to piracetam (at doses of only 800mg) that I decided to give her a small raise so she could afford it. She takes piracetam instead of heading for the coffee machine. Every day she takes it she is decidedly more alert, and intelligent-acting and she smiles more. She is overall a much better employee. She says it wakes up her brain." —JM

"Piracetam keeps me alert when I am driving. It also helps me to formulate new and different ideas when I am taking essay tests in school."—DB

"I liked piracetam so much that I decided to try it with vincamine and xanthinol nicotinate. I took standard doses of all three - 2400mg of piracetam, 20mg of vincamine and 300mg of xanthinol nicotinate. I actually felt stupid! I had the "right on the tip of my tongue" response for hours.

Recently a friend suggested that I combine Hydergine with piracetam, explaining that the two synergize each other, and that I should try a small dose of each. I had tried Hydergine years ago and liked it a lot, but found it prohibitively expensive. I decided to experiment with these two in combination with ginkgo biloba. I started with what I thought were very small quantities, 1/4mg of Hydergine, 200mg of piracetam, and 50mg of ginkgo, but found the combination to be extraordinary. I've tried many different smart drugs and nutrients, but this low-cost, low-dose combination is my favorite."—BP

"I started taking piracetam with choline about a year ago and have found this combination to be one of the best things that ever happened to me. I no longer get extreme mood swings, I am much happier in general, and my concentration and speaking ability is better. I also found that my relationships with family and friends have improved, probably due to my increased self-confidence."—HH

"I took two grams of piracetam and, after 30 minutes, I began to find my boyfriend much more sexually attractive. I assumed this was a fluke since I had never heard of this effect from piracetam. Since this experience I have taken piracetam every day for two months and every time, without fail, it has had the same effect. Piracetam has vastly improved my sex life."—DB

"Intelligence is the ultimate aphrodisiac."—Tim Leary

Pyroglutamate:

"I have discovered that I really enjoy using PCA during the daytime since it helps me to feel focused and clear when I work. I have found that a teaspoon of PCA mixed in a glass of juice tastes best and gives me a healthy alternative to my usual morning coffee. The most beneficial effects to me are the increased alertness and ability to concentrate so much better."—DB

"I am 66 years old and work as a writer, so my ability to formulate new thoughts is especially important. When I took one teaspoon of PCA I began to wake up and I could feel my mind begin to click right along at a faster pace. After two hours a few friends stopped by, so I quickly became engaged in a conversation that might otherwise have been difficult to keep up with. But this time there was something distinctly different about my own contribution to the conversation, for I noticed that the things that I had to say were witty and logical. It took me a while to figure out why I felt so differently, and then I realized it was the PCA."—GB

Centrophenoxine:

"I had been having a problem with fatigue and depression which disappeared when I started taking centrophenoxine. Centrophenoxine also improved my memory and made me much quicker."—JC

DMAE:

"A few years ago I tried a precursor of acetylcholine called DMAE. I loved the effects. When I did a little research I found that acetylcholine was the brain chemical that was inhibited by car sickness medications. I already knew that taking too many Dramamines caused one to be unable to distinguish between fantasy and reality. This fit my experience perfectly: when I take DMAE, I am more awake when I am awake, more sound asleep when I am asleep. Not only does my memory improve, but I have an easier time daydreaming when I want to, and concentrating on real-world tasks when I want to."—BP

Hydergine:

"I first tried Hydergine six years ago with some fascinating results. During a visit to see my Dad at Christmas, he and I started taking 9mg per day of Hydergine in the hope it would help to improve our long-term memory. The results were apparent to us both within two days. He was in his 40's, and could remember events from when he was in his 20's. They were as clear in his mind as if they happened yesterday. The events were family vacations, picnics, and holidays. What was unique about these memories was that the events weren't especially outstanding times. So in other words, the everyday events truly had been stored away all these years, it just took some chemical prodding to jog them loose into the conscious mind. I was in my early 20's and my memories went back to the childhood years. A unique opportunity had been presented to us to sit down and really share in the joys that our life had brought us. What a gift!"—DB

Propranolol:

"I have always had a terrible problem with stage fright. For years I played music alone in my room, and when I danced I did it alone with the shades drawn. While dancing, the slightest bump in the hallway outside my apartment could make me freeze with an immobilizing adrenaline rush. I read about propranolol and asked my doctor for it immediately. He had heard of this use for propranolol and gave me a few tablets to try. I began to play music while using it, alone at first, then with others. With each successive experience it became easier and easier. I used propranolol while dancing and then began to go out to clubs. I soon discovered that once I had used propranolol three or four times in a particular club I no longer needed it. Now the effects have generalized to all my dancing and playing music, unless I am playing with new musicians. I still use propranolol for job interviews, first dates (although I recently forgot and didn't notice until the next day), and any other fear-producing situation."—BP

Vasopressin:

"The most immediate result from using Vasopressin is the increased clarity and alertness. I can be logical without the usual speediness associated with caffeine use. After five minutes I've noticed that I'm busily accomplishing tasks that I'd been putting off for a week. The duration is about two hours for the energetic feelings. Overall, I feel my short-term memory recall improving over the past two weeks of using Vasopressin. It seems that the longer I use it, the more I can rely on my mind to be a portable note pad."—DB

"Being a student is less stressful now that I have Vasopressin to use. I can count on my mind being clear enough to formulate test answers, even if I feel tired or foggy-headed."—DB

"During my final year as an undergraduate I decided to change majors from psychology to mathematics. I was also running out of money and I knew I had to finish in one year and then get a job. I started using a combination of Hydergine, vasopressin, pemoline, and a good vitamin formula with large amounts of choline. This particular combination improved my concentration enormously. I flew through that year taking a full load of upper level mathematics courses each semester. Not only did I complete the major in the allotted time, but my grades were better than I was used to. I was getting As instead of Bs. I landed a job in Silicon Valley immediately after graduation. In other words, everything went perfectly according to plan and I really don't think I could have done it without the smart drugs."—SR

Appendix E:
Sources For Further Information

The Age Reduction System, Dr.Richard Kaufman, 1986, published by Rawson Associates, New York, N.Y.

This very-well-researched book covers much basic information about life extension.

A Remarkable Medicine Has Been Overlooked, Jack Dreyfus, 1981, published by Simon and Schuster, New York, NY.

This painstakingly-researched book is the fruit of Dreyfus' 20-year effort to alert the medical profession and the world at large to the benefits of phenytoin (Dilantin). The book has a great 2140-reference bibliography and review that covers some of the most important discoveries about this incredible drug.

Biological Aging Measurement: Clinical Applications, Ward Dean, M.D., 1988, published by The Center for Bio-Gerontology, P.O. Box 11097, Pensacola, FL 32524.

"... *A valuable reference ... the first time that anyone has seriously proposed the use of these systems to measure the aging processes.*"—Johan Bjorksten, Ph.D.

"... *Highly recommended for anyone involved in anti-aging therapy or experimentation.*"—Roy Walford, M.D.

"... *The most pertinent life extension book available.*"—John A. Mann.

This book is designed for biomedical gerontologists and life-extension experimenters to evaluate the efficacy of experimental life extension/age retarding programs. It describes over 200 physiological, biochemical and psychometric parameters that change with age.

The Complete Guide to Anti-Aging Nutrients, by Sheldon Saul Hendler, M.D., published by Simon and Schuster.

This is a very comprehensive, even-handed evaluation of nearly every nutrient purported to have anti-aging effects. It is encyclopedic and provides a wealth of scientific references.

Dialog Information Services, 3460 Hillview Ave., Palo Alto, CA 94304, Phone: (415) 858 2700.

Dialog is the world's largest online information service. This means that people use their computers to call Dialog and search hundreds of databases for answers to their questions. Dialog is expensive and takes some time to learn to use, but it offers a sister service called Knowledge Index that is much easier to search and is available during non-business hours at a reduced cost of $24 per hour. Much of the research we did to write this book was done by conducting more than a hundred searches of MedLine (the online version of the National Library of Medicine) with Knowledge Index.

If you have been diagnosed as having a disease and want to know about the latest treatment research or if you want to know about the research on a particular drug you can have a search of MedLine (or any other online database) done by a reference librarian at many libraries. There are also companies who will conduct an online search for you for a fee, including Life Services Supplements at (800) 542 3230.

Drugs Available Abroad, Jerry L. Schlesser, Ed., and Derwent Publications Ltd., 1991, published by Gale Research Inc., Detroit, MI.

Covers over 1000 drugs that are approved in other countries but not approved in the United States. Contains hard-to-find therapeutic information, drug action, precautions, dosage, etc.

Forefront-Health Investigations (formerly Journal of the MegaHealth Society), Editor: Steven Wm. Fowkes, six-issue subscription $18 (third class mail), $21 (first class mail), $21 (Canadian), $25 (overseas airmail), P.O. Box 60637, Palo Alto, CA 94306, Phone: (408) 733 2010.

This newsletter reviews medical technologies rarely covered anywhere else. While oriented towards life extension, the journal goes far afield to cover the work of the likes of Emanuel Revici (the New York physician responsible for a whole theory of biology based on the body's acid and alkaline balance), alternative cancer treatments, chelation therapy and political issues. The writing is excellent and easy to understand.

How to Live Longer and Feel Better, Linus Pauling, 1986, published by W. H. Freeman, New York, NY.

Pauling is the two-time Nobel Prize winning biochemist who has been reviled by the medical establishment for his research into the health benefits of vitamin C and other antioxidants. If one talks to Pauling's peers, that is, actual scientists rather than medical doctors, a different picture appears: Crick and Watson credit Pauling with the co-discovery of the structure of DNA. Pauling would probably have shared Crick and Watson's Nobel Prize had he been able to join them in their research. However, he was denied travel visas during the McCarthy era due to his pacifist beliefs and activities. A reporter researching Pauling for Penthouse magazine in the late '80s talked to many of the top physicists and biochemists in the U.S. and found they all agreed; Pauling is one of the greatest minds our country has produced.

How to Live Longer and Feel Better outlines Pauling's personal life extension program and includes 30 pages of scientific references, easy-to-understand explanations of the mechanisms of aging and the actions of vitamins, and the eye-opening story of the "controversy" about vitamins.

Life Extension, A Practical Scientific Approach, Durk Pearson and Sandy Shaw, 1982, published by Warner Books, New York, NY.

Pearson and Shaw made the term "life extension" a household word with their best-seller, their many television appearances and their incredible recall of the research and its implications.

This 858-page book addresses all aspects of aging, including sexuality, cancer, heart attack risk reduction, intelligence increase, and depression. Written in a friendly and sometimes humorous style, *Life Extension* has practical "how-to" type suggestions for slowing down the rate of aging in your own body, all based on scientific research.

The book is fun to read, and also makes a great reference manual. It's designed to be used by both professional people and non-professionals. *Life Extension* has an excellent index, and many health problems or questions are listed with several pages to which you can refer.

Pearson and Shaw delayed publication of *Life Extension* for a year because Warner Books thought that the 96 pages of scientific references were unnecessary. Warner Books relented to avoid the law suit that the authors initiated to insure the inclusion of their bibliography. Obviously, the science behind their work is important to Sandy and Durk.

Mind Food and Smart Pills, Ross Pelton, R.Ph., Ph.D. with Taffy Clark Pelton, 1989, published by Doubleday, New York, NY 10103.

This book presents a compendium of vitamins, herbs, and drugs that can work wonders for the human mind. From antioxidants like Vitamin C and selenium that counteract the damaging effects of free radicals, to herbs such as ginseng and Ginkgo biloba that can combat brain aging, each supplement is covered in detail.

The Neuroendocrine Theory of Aging and Degenerative Disease, by Vladimir M. Dilman, M.D., Ph.D., D.M.Sc., and Ward Dean, M.D., published by the Center for Bio-Gerontology, P.O. Box 11097, Pensacola, FL 32524.

Professor Dilman is one of the most widely known scientists in the Soviet Union. Dilman theorizes that aging is a disease that everyone over the age of 30 "catches", and that all of the other age-related conditions are merely symptoms of this one "super-disease". The book proposes unique therapeutic regimens to delay the onset of aging and treat age-related diseases.

Orphan Drugs, Kenneth Anderson and Lois Anderson, 1987, published by The Body Press, Los Angeles, CA 90048.

Orphan Drugs is a "Physicians' Desk Reference" for over 1500 drugs that are available outside the U.S., but for various reasons have not been "adopted" by U.S. pharmaceutical companies. The Andersons include two separate indexes, one for the various trade and chemical names under which the drugs are sold, and one for the symptoms and diseases that the drugs are used to treat. There is a great directory of drug manufacturers, and the book also has an excellent description of how the FDA works (and doesn't work) in this country.

Physicians' Desk Reference, annual, published by Medical Economics Company, Oradell, NJ.

This is a guide for physicians to the use of drugs that the Food and Drug Administration approves for use in the U.S. Only FDA-approved drug uses are listed here, and this book is the sole source of information about pharmaceuticals for many physicians. You can find the PDR in most libraries. Each drug's listing includes contraindications, dosage information, drug interactions, and adverse effects.

Physicians Guide to Free Radicals, Immunity and Aging, by Lord Lee-Benner, M.D., published by the World Health Foundation, 360 San Miguel Drive, Suite 208, Newport Beach, CA 92660. Tel: (714) 720 9022.

This book is a comprehensive explanation of how free radicals contribute to cancer, atherosclerosis, and the diseases of aging. Lee-Benner gives special emphasis to Alzheimer's disease and how it develops. The book includes specific dietary, nutritional and pharmacological prescriptions for delaying the onset of aging and reversing age-related conditions.

Smart Drug News, $40 per year (10 issue) subscription. CERI, P.O. Box 4029-2009, Menlo Park, CA 94026-4029.

Published by the Cognition Enhancement Research Institute (CERI), this is a newsletter devoted exclusively to covering the latest smart drug and nutrient research. In the letters-to-the-editor section, consumers can get their questions answered by experts on smart drugs.

Appendix F: FDA Drug Bulletin

The appropriateness or the legality of prescribing approved drugs for uses not included in their official labeling is sometimes a cause of concern and confusion among practitioners.

Under the federal Food, Drug, and Cosmetic (FD&C) Act, a drug approved for marketing may be labeled, promoted, and advertised by the manufacturer only for those uses for which the drug's safety and effectiveness have been established and which the FDA has approved. These are commonly referred to as "approved uses". This means that adequate and well-controlled clinical trials have documented these uses, and the results of the trials have been reviewed and approved by the FDA.

The FD&C Act does not, however, limit the manner in which a physician may use an approved drug. Once a product has been approved for marketing, a physician may prescribe it for uses or in treatment regimens or patient populations that are not included in approved labeling. Such "unapproved" uses may be appropriate and rational in certain circumstances, and may, in fact, reflect approaches to drug therapy that have been extensively reported in medical literature.

The term "unapproved uses" is, to some extent, misleading. It includes a variety of situations ranging from unstudied to thoroughly investigated drug uses. Valid new uses for drugs already on the market are often first discovered through serendipitous observations and therapeutic innovations, subsequently confirmed by well-planned and executed clinical investigation. Before such advances can be added to the approved labeling, however, data substantiating the effectiveness of a new use or regimen must be submitted by the manufacturer to the FDA for evaluation. This may take time and, without the initiative of the drug manufacturer whose product is involved, may never occur. For that reason, accepted medical practice often includes drug use that is not reflected in approved drug labeling.

With respect to its role in medical practice, the package insert is informational only. The FDA tries to assure that prescription drug information in the package insert accurately and fully reflects the data on safety and effectiveness on which drug approval is based.

193

Appendix G:
FDA Policy on Mail Importations

DATE: JULY 20, 1988

FROM: DIRECTOR, OFFICE OF REGIONAL OPERATIONS (HFC-100)

SUBJ: "PILOT GUIDANCE FOR RELEASE OF MAIL IMPORTATIONS"

TO : REGIONAL FOOD AND DRUG DIRECTORS
      DISTRICT DIRECTORS
      IMPORT PROGRAM MANAGERS
      COMPLIANCE BRANCH DIRECTORS
      INVESTIGATIONS BRANCH DIRECTORS
      LABORATORY BRANCH DIRECTORS

INFO: ALL MAJOR FIELD OFFICES

* * * * * * * * * * CORRECTED COPY * * * * * *
NOTE: THIS GUIDANCE IS BEING ISSUED ON A PILOT BASIS AND IS SUBJECT TO CHANGE AND/OR CANCELLATION, IF THE PILOT PROVES SUCCESSFUL, WITH NO SIGNIFICANT PROBLEMS, CHAPTER 9-71 OF THE REGULATORY PROCEDURES MANUAL MAY BE APPROPRIATELY REVISED.

SUBJ: Pilot Guidance for Release of Mail Importations

Because of the desire to acquire articles for treatment of serious and life-threatening conditions like AIDS and cancer, individuals have been purchasing unapproved products from foreign sources. Some of these products are sold over-the-counter in the country of origin while others are available from clinics where the purchaser was treated. Such products are often shipped to the purchaser by mail.

Even though such products are subject to refusal, we may use our discretion to examine the background, risk, and purpose of these products before making a final decision. To assure that the districts are operating in a uniform manner, the following guidance is provided for dealing with personal use shipments.

1. Except as modified by these instructions, established guidance found in RPM-9-71, exhibits X9-71-1 and X9-71-2 should be followed.

2. A product entered for personal use, which meets the criteria in item 4 below, may proceed without sampling or detention.

3. Products that are not identified, or are not accompanied by documentation of intended use, should be detained. Other reasons for detention may include: size of the shipment (amount inconsistent with personal use), fraudulent promotion or misrepresentation, or an unreasonable health risk due to either toxicity or possible contamination. In such cases, the appropriate center should be contacted for guidance concerning release of the product.

4. Following detention, shipments may be released to an individual if the following criteria can be satisfied and there is no safety risk or evidence of fraud:

   * the product was purchased for personal use.

   * the product is not for commercial distribution and the amount of product is not excessive (i.e., 3 months supply of a drug).

   * the intended use of the product is appropriately identified.

   * the patient seeking to import the product affirms in writing that it is for the patient's own use and provides the name and address of the doctor licensed in the U.S. responsible for his or her treatment with the product.

5. If the district should encounter a situation suggesting promotional and/or commercial activity that falls within our health fraud guideline, the district should recommend that an Import Alert be issued for the automatic detention of the product and identification of the promoter involved.

6. The model letter currently in Exhibit X9-71-2 should be revised according to the attached during this pilot.

7. The article may then be RELEASED WITH COMMENT upon receipt of the

letter as follows:

> "The drug you have obtained for your personal use appears to be unapproved in the U.S. We understand you will use this limited quantity under medical supervision; however, future personal shipments may be refused entry if we learn, among other things, the drug presents an unreasonable risk or it has been commercially promoted to U.S. citizens."

The above guidance should be used as part of the current outstanding instructions for dealing with mail packages as found in Chapter 9-71 or the RPM.

Ronald G. Chesemore

9-70-00 <u>PURPOSE</u>

This chapter provides guidance for special procedures covering certain specific commodities and problems. Surveys have shown a significant variance among the districts in the area. A typical example is the district's coverage of mail importations which varies from 0% to 100%. Such unequal enforcement is unfair to both the consuming public and the trade.

If there is a need for additional guidance in this area, the Assistant for Import Operations in EDRO/Field Compliance Branch (HFO-110) should be contacted.

It should be noted that FDA has entered into agreements with a number of foreign countries including Belgium, Canada, France, Netherlands, and Mexico for cooperation and exchange of information. Some of these agreements may have an impact on our import coverage; consequently, the involved districts should be aware of the various provisions therein. These agreements are published as memos of Understanding in Chapter 55, Compliance Policy Guides Manual.

9-71-00 <u>PURPOSE</u>

To provide general guidance for the coverage of imports entered through the mails so as to provide the greatest degree of public protection within allotted resources.

9-71-10 <u>BACKGROUND</u>

We know that it is easy to spend much time and effort covering mail importations just as it is covering importations in personal baggage. However, again as with imports in personal baggage, coverage of mail importations results in little consumer protection because the transactions are personal and are small, both in size and value. We must remember the consumer protection provided by unlimited, extensive coverage of mail imports is not commensurate with the resources that are expended.

Some districts appear to be expending relatively more resources than others on the coverage of mail importations. This type of program can be ineffective in terms of the best consumer protection that can be provided.

9-71-20 <u>OBJECTIVES</u>

A.   To adjust the attention given coverage of mail importations.

B.   To provide a balanced and uniform approach for the coverage of mail imports.

C.   To provide the greatest degree of public protection within allotted resources.

D.   To affirm FDA's policy regarding the coverage of mail importations.

9-71-30 GUIDANCE

Generally, little time should be spent on the coverage of mail importations. Articles entering through the mails should not be detained except for the following substantial reasons:

A. When the size of the packages(s) (lot) or the number of entries from a particular shipper or to a specific addressee in a given time period indicates the merchandise may be for commercial instead of personal use.

B. Importations (articles) which present an imminent danger to health.

C. When an "Import Alert" has been issued concerning a specific commodity.

D. When importations (articles), brought to our attention, are clearly actionable such as new drugs that are not covered by an approved NDA.

9-71-40 PROCESSING PROCEDURES FOR MAIL IMPORTATIONS

Generally, the procedure for handling mail importations should be the following:

— Parcels should be opened and examined by the Customs Mail Division. Those believed to be subject to one or more of the criteria above should be set aside for examination by FDA.

— Complete the Form FD-725 "Mail Collection Report" for each parcel selected for sampling. Generally a physical sample is not required on mail importations because a documentary sample e.g., labels, inserts, etc., will be sufficient for most label violations. However, if a physical sample is needed collect only the amount needed for analysis by the laboratory from the mail parcel. The remaining portion should not be removed from the custody of the U.S. Customs mail Division.

— Violative mail importations detained according to the above listed criteria should be held by U.S. Customs in the mail room until either released or refused entry.

— Attached as guides are two specimen letters that may be sent with the Notice of Detention and Hearing when a parcel is detained.

> Exhibit X9-71-1 - for use in general mail importations.

> Exhibit X9-71-2 - for use in prescription drug mail importations.

— Articles not subject to the FD&C Act but are contained with items subject to the Act should be listed on the mail collection report in the event of any question regarding the contents of the parcel at a later date.

— If the consignee submits a request for the release of those items not subject to FDA jurisdiction in a detained mail importation, and the request is accompanied with a statement permitting destruction of the violative article, the request with the statement and a Notice of Refusal of Admission covering the violative article should be referred to the Mail Division of U.S. Customs having custody of the parcel so they can determine final disposition of all merchandise, including destruction of the violative portion.

Model Letter for Use in General Mail Importations
Exhibit X9-71-1
==

(LETTERHEAD)

A mail shipment of an article from a foreign country addressed to you is being detained at the post office. All products of this kind must meet the requirements of the Federal Food, Drug, and Cosmetic Act of the other Acts enforced by FDA. These laws are designed to protect you from unsafe or misrepresented foods, drugs, cosmetics, devices, and other articles. Examination indicates the product addressed to you does not comply with the law.

Please read the enclosed Notice of Detention and Hearing carefully since it explains why the product is believed to be in violation. The notice does not in any manner accuse you of violating any law.

If you have good reason to believe the product does comply with the law and wish to discuss it with us, you may come personally to this office or write to us within the time limit shown on the Notice.

If you do not wish to do this, you may disregard the Notice.

The product will be returned to the sender without cost to you if we do not hear from you within the time stated.

Sincerely yours,

Model Letter for Use in Prescription Drug Mail
Exhibit X9-71-2

===

(LETTERHEAD)

A mail shipment of an article from a foreign country addressed to you is being detained at the post office. All products of this kind must meet the requirements of the Federal Food, Drug, and Cosmetic Act, which is designed to protect you from unsafe or misrepresented foods, drugs, cosmetics and devices. Examination indicates the product addressed to you does not comply with the law.

Please read the enclosed Notice of Detention and Hearing carefully since it explains why the product is believed to be in violation. The notice does not in any manner accuse you of violating any law.

If this drug is not an investigational or new drug and you are taking it under the supervision of a physician, it may be released for your use provided you furnish the following:

> 1. A written statement from your physician (licensed by law to practice medicine in the United States), requesting that the drug be delivered to him for your use under his supervision.

> 2. A written statement from you, addressed to the post office authorizing them to readdress the package to your physician (Give his name and office address).

Send both statements to this office, and we will make arrangements promptly for release of the product.

If you have good reason to believe the product does comply with the law and wish to discuss it with us, you may come personally to this office or write to us within the time limit shown on the Notice. If you do not wish to do this, you may disregard the Notice.

The product will be returned to the sender without cost to you if we do not hear from you within the time stated.

Sincerely yours,

Glossary

Acetylcholine (ACh): A neurotransmitter which plays an important role in memory. It is also used for control of sensory input signals and muscular control. ACh is a stimulatory neurotransmitter. When released by muscle nerves, it makes those muscles contract. It is made from the precursor nutrient choline and there is some evidence that increased dietary choline can increase production and use of acetylcholine. Also, many drugs affect the production and release of this neurotransmitter.

Age Pigment: (See lipofuscin).

Alzheimer's disease: Also called SDAT (senile dementia Alzheimer's type). This disease is characterized by a general loss of intellectual ability and impairment of memory, judgment, and abstract thinking as well as changes in personality. Other symptoms include loss of speech, disorientation, and apathy. Alzheimer's disease is the most common cause of dementia, rarely occurring before the age of 50. The disease takes from a few months to four or five years to progress to complete loss of intellectual function.

Amino Acid: an organic acid containing an amine (ammonia-like) chemical group. Amino acids are put together by your body in highly specific ways to manufacture proteins.

Antioxidant: a nutrient or chemical that reacts with and neutralizes free radicals or chemicals that release free radicals. Antioxidants are also called free radical scavengers. Vitamins A, C, E, some of the B vitamins, beta-carotene, selenium, and some key enzymes in your body are all antioxidants. By intercepting the free radicals, antioxidants prevent them from damaging delicate molecular structures such as your DNA. See Free Radicals.

ATP: Adenosine triphosphate, the universal energy molecule, created in the mitochondria of your cells using energy derived from the food you eat. All the cellular activities in your body use the energy released by splitting ATP.

Catecholamines: the class of neurotransmitters that includes norepinephrine, and dopamine.

Central Nervous System (CNS): the brain, spinal cord, and their associated nerves.

Cerebrovascular Insufficiency: an inadequate supply of blood to the brain because of a narrowing of the blood vessels which lead to, or are in various areas of the brain.

Cholinergic: the parts of the nervous system that use acetylcholine as a neurotransmitter.

Dendrites: the fine network of branches that extend from the body of a nerve cell, receiving impulses and carrying them into the center of the cell.

DNA: deoxyribonucleic acid, the genetic blueprint that resides in the nucleus of every cell of every living organism ever studied. Many researchers believe that free radical damage to the DNA is directly involved in aging and cancer.

Dopamine: a neurotransmitter critical to fine motor coordination, immune function, motivation, insulin regulation, physical energy, thinking, short-term memory, emotions such as sexual desire, and autonomic nervous system balance.

Dopaminergic: the parts of the nervous system which use dopamine as a neurotransmitter.

Double-Blind: a type of scientific experiment in which neither the subjects nor the researchers know who is receiving an active substance and who is receiving a placebo. The data generated from the experiment is then usually evaluated by researchers who do not know which subjects received the active substance. This type of experiment helps to eliminate personal bias from research.

Double-Blind Crossover: a double-blind study where at one point in the experiment all of the subjects switch from an active substance to a placebo or vice versa.

Free Radical: a highly chemically reactive atom, molecule or molecular fragment with a free or unpaired electron. Free radicals are produced in many different ways such as: normal metabolic processes, ultraviolet radiation from the sun, nuclear radiation, and the breakdown in the body of spoiled fats. Free radicals have been implicated in aging, cancer, cardiovascular disease, and other kinds of damage to the body. See Antioxidants.

Free-Radical Reaction: the cascade of chemical reactions that occurs when a free radical reacts with another molecule in order to gain an electron. The molecule that loses an electron to the free radical then becomes a free radical, repeating the process until the energy of the free radical is spent or the reaction is stopped by an antioxidant. In biological systems this cascade can damage important molecules like DNA.

GABA: gamma aminobutyric acid, an amino acid which acts as an inhibitory neurotransmitter.

Growth Hormone (GH): a hormone secreted by the pituitary gland. GH stimulates growth and repair of the body as well as the activities of the immune system. With age, GH release diminishes.

Hormone: a chemical messenger such as growth hormone, testosterone or insulin.

Hypoxia: a condition of lowered oxygen levels in the blood. Hypoxia promotes free-radical activity in the body.

Inhibitory neurotransmitter: a neurotransmitter which decreases the electro-chemical activity of neurons. GABA (gamma aminobutyric acid) and serotonin are inhibitory neurotransmitters.

Learning: a change in neural function as a consequence of experience.

Lipofuscin: the brown waste material deposited in skin and nerve cells that is commonly called "age spots." Lipofuscin is made of free-radical-damaged proteins and fats.

Liver spots: deposits of lipofuscin in skin.

Monamine oxidase (MAO): an enzyme which, in the brain, breaks down certain neurotransmitters such as serotonin, dopamine, and norepinephrine.

Nerve: a cell which carries information to and from the central nervous system.

Nerve Growth Factor (NGF): a naturally occurring hormone that stimulates the growth of neurites.

Neurites: the tiny projections growing from each nerve cell which carries information between the cells. A nerve cell may have over 100,000 neurites growing out of it, each connected to another nerve cell.

Neurochemical: a chemical that naturally occurs in the nervous system and plays a part in its functioning.

Neuron: a nerve cell.

Neurotransmitter: one of the many chemicals that carries impulses between nerve cells.

Nootropic: a word coined by Dr. Giurgea to describe a new class of drugs that act as cognitive enhancers with no side effects or toxicity, from the Greek words noos, meaning mind and tropein meaning toward. (See the section on Nootropics.)

Norepinephrine: an excitatory neurotransmitter involved in alertness, concentration, aggression and motivation, among other behaviors. Norepinephrine is made in the brain from the amino acid phenylalanine.

Oxidation: a chemical reaction in which an electron is taken from a molecule of the oxidized substance.

Parkinson's disease: a chronic disease of the central nervous system caused by lowered levels of the inhibitory neurotransmitter dopamine. Symptoms include muscular tremors and weakness.

Pituitary gland: a gland at the base of the brain. The pituitary secretes several different hormones involved in key metabolic processes.

Placebo: an inert compound usually given to a portion of the subjects in a scientific experiment in order to distinguish the psychological effects of the experiment from the physiological effects of the drug being tested.

Precursor: a chemical which can be converted by the body into another is a precursor of the latter chemical.

Receptors: sites on the outside of cells where particular messenger molecules such as hormones can attach. This attachment to the receptor site causes corresponding changes inside the cell.

Regeneration: the regrowth of cells, tissues, organs, or limbs.

Senility: the aging-related loss of mental faculties.

Serotonin: an inhibitory neurotransmitter required for sleep.

Stimulatory Neurotransmitter: a neurotransmitter that increases electro-chemical activity in the nerve cells. Norepinephrine is an stimulatory neurotransmitter.

Stroke: a rupture in a blood vessel in the brain, often with disastrous effects depending on where the rupture occurs.

Synergy: when compounds are combined and their effects are more than the sum of their individual effects, the compounds are said to have positive synergy. Many of the compounds we write about here have positive synergistic effects with each other.

Systemic: throughout the entire body.

Toxic: poisonous. Everything, including water and oxygen, is toxic in sufficiently high doses.

Index

211

About The Authors

Ward Dean, M.D., has been actively engaged in geronto-logical research for over 10 years, and has published more than 50 articles and reviews in professional journals. He is the medical director of the Center for Bio-Gerontology in Pensacola, Florida. Dr. Dean is the author of *Biological Aging Measurement*, published in 1988, and co-author, with Professor Vladimir Dilman, of *The Neuroendocrine Theory of Aging and Degenerative Disease*.

John Morgenthaler is a science writer in Santa Cruz, California. He has degrees in psychology and computer science and has worked in the field of artificial intelligence. John has been researching smart drugs & nutrients since 1980.